# *Wall Pilates for Weight Loss*

# Disclaimer

Before beginning any exercise program or following the directions in this book, it is strongly recommended that you consult a physician or exercise professional.

The author and publishers of this book are not responsible for any injury or damage resulting from the use or interpretation of the information provided.

Please keep in mind that each person is unique and has different levels of physical condition and health. It is essential to listen to your body, avoid pushing yourself beyond your limits, and adapt the exercises according to your personal abilities and condition.

The proposed exercises may involve risks, and it is necessary to perform them appropriately and responsibly.

Make sure to perform the exercises in a safe and appropriate environment, using stable and suitable equipment.

# Mission of the Book

Welcome to the wonderful world of Pilates on the wall! In this book, I introduce myself, Eden Stone, as a passionate fitness author and an expert guide in achieving your weight loss goals through this fascinating discipline.

Have you ever wanted a workout method that is effective for weight loss and allows you to exercise in the comfort of your own home? Pilates on a wall is the answer. Over the course of these pages, I will take you on a journey of physical and mental transformation, sharing with you the strategies, secrets, and training programs I have developed during my years of experience.

But why Pilates on a wall? First of all, it is important to understand that Pilates itself is a comprehensive discipline, involving both body and mind. It is a method that aims to develop muscle strength, improve flexibility, increase body awareness, and promote mental balance. But when we combine Pilates with wall support, new possibilities open up.

Pilates on a wall offers many benefits that make it ideal for those who wish to lose weight. By using the wall as a point of reference and resistance, you will experience greater stability and control during exercises. This will allow you to work on different parts of your body in a focused way, engaging your deep muscles and boosting your endurance. In addition, the wall support will help you maintain proper posture and perform the exercises safely and effectively.

Through Pilates on the wall, you will have the opportunity to work your entire body, toning muscles, improving balance and flexibility, and burning calories effectively. But that's not all: wall Pilates will allow you to strengthen your core, stabilizing your spine and improving your overall posture.

In this book, I will guide you step by step, offering detailed instructions and clear illustrations for each exercise. I will be your traveling companion, providing support, motivation, and practical advice to help you achieve your weight loss goals.

If you are ready to embark on this journey of physical and mental transformation, then it's time to get started. I am here for you, ready to accompany you on your wall Pilates adventure and provide all the support you need.

Get ready to discover a new dimension of fitness with Pilates on the wall and embrace a life full of health and wellness.

# CONTENTS

# INTRODUCTION

Pilates on the wall is a fascinating variation of traditional Pilates that combines the fundamental elements of Pilates with the use of the wall as a benchmark and resistance point. This innovative approach offers numerous benefits for those seeking to lose weight and improve their overall well-being.

Wall Pilates is based on the basic principles of traditional Pilates, including:

- Control:
  Movement control is essential in wall Pilates. Exercises are performed in a controlled and mindful manner, focusing on proper body alignment and correct execution of movements.

- Breathing:
  Breathing is an integral part of Pilates on the wall. Deep, mindful breathing helps stabilize the core and maintain a steady flow of oxygen during exercises.

- Core:
  In Pilates on a wall, work on the "core" of the body, simply known as the core, is crucial. The core includes the abdominal, lumbar, and pelvic muscles, which provide a solid foundation of stability for the rest of the body.

- Fluidity and precision:
  Wall Pilates exercises are characterized by fluid, controlled, and precise movements. The goal is to perform the exercises with grace and precision, avoiding abrupt movements or excessive effort.

- Concentration and awareness:
  In wall Pilates, concentration and awareness are crucial. During exercises, it is important to be present and focused on body sensations, alignment, and correct execution of movements.

Pilates on a wall offers a number of unique benefits for those wishing to lose weight. By using the wall as a reference point, greater stability and control can be achieved during exercises, engaging deep muscles and working on different parts of the body in a targeted manner. The wall's support promotes correct posture, reduces the risk of injury, and allows you to perform exercises safely and effectively.

In addition, Pilates on the wall helps tone muscles, improve balance and flexibility, and burn calories effectively. Through the specific exercises of Pilates on the wall, you can strengthen your core, stabilize your spine, and improve your overall posture.

Pilates on a wall is a versatile and accessible option for people of different ages and fitness levels. It is suitable for both beginners and experts, as the exercises can be adapted to different individual abilities.

With Pilates on a wall, you have the opportunity to discover a new dimension of fitness that will help you achieve your weight loss goals and improve your overall well-being.

Another fascinating feature of Pilates on a wall is its versatility. You can customize the exercises to suit your individual needs and abilities. Whether you are a beginner looking to build a solid foundation of strength and flexibility or an expert looking for new challenges, Pilates on the wall offers a wide range of variations and progressions that will allow you to progress gradually.

In addition to traditional wall Pilates, there are other variations you can explore. For example, Pilates on a wall with the use of additional equipment, such as elastic bands or balls, can add variety and resistance to your workouts. You can even combine Pilates on a wall with other disciplines, such as yoga or cardio training, to create customized programs that meet your specific weight loss and wellness needs.

Get ready to discover a new perspective on fitness and transform your body and mind through Pilates on the wall. I am excited to accompany you on this journey of positive change for a better life.

# PREPARATION FOR PILATES ON A WALL

## Tools and Equipment

Practicing Pilates on a wall requires the use of some specific tools and equipment that will enable you to perform the exercises safely and effectively. Here is an overview of the tools and equipment needed:

- Mat:
  A yoga mat or any other soft mat is essential to provide adequate cushioning during exercises. Be sure to choose a good-quality mat that is thick enough to protect your back and joints during exercise.

- Wall:
  The wall becomes your main reference point during wall Pilates. Make sure you have adequate space with a solid wall and no sharp or protruding objects that could cause damage or hinder movement.

- Elastic band or strap:
  An elastic band or strap can be used to add resistance and variety to exercises. These tools can be clipped to the wall or used to stabilize specific parts of the body while performing exercises. Be sure to use a good-quality elastic band or strap that provides the right amount of resistance for your fitness level.

- Pilates ball or fitball:
  The Pilates ball, or fitball, is a versatile piece of equipment that can be used to perform a variety of Pilates exercises on a wall. It can be used to increase balance, stability, and intensity of exercises. Be sure to choose an appropriately sized ball based on your height and personal preferences.

- Pillows or back supports:
  Depending on your comfort level and personal needs, you may opt to use back pillows or supports during exercises. These can provide extra support and comfort, especially for those who have back problems or seek extra support during movement.

- Comfortable and suitable clothing:
  Wearing comfortable and appropriate clothing is essential while practicing Pilates on a wall. Opt for clothing that allows you to move freely and does not restrict movement. Be sure to wear sneakers or comfortable shoes that provide support and stability during the exercises.

Make sure you have all the tools and equipment you need before you start your Pilates on the wall workout. This will allow you to perform the exercises safely and effectively, maximizing the benefits and achieving significant results.

# Adapting the Training Environment

The beauty of Pilates on a wall is that it can be practiced in the comfort of your own home, without the need for a gym or expensive equipment. However, it is important to prepare a proper workout environment to maximize the benefits and ensure safety while performing the exercises. Here are some suggestions for adapting your workout environment at home:

- Dedicated space:
  Dedicate a specific space for practicing Pilates on a wall. Choose an area that has enough room to move freely and without obstacles. To create a pleasant and motivating environment, make sure it is well lit and ventilated.

- Cleanliness and safety:
  Before starting the workout, make sure the area is clean and free of objects that could cause injury. Remove any slippery carpets or fragile objects that could be damaged during exercises. To avoid accidents, make sure the floor is stable and not slippery.

- Wall bracket:
  Check that the wall you will be practicing on is solid and strong. Avoid using walls with brittle or damaged siding. Also, if you plan to use tools such as elastic bands or straps, make sure the wall can withstand the tension generated by these tools.

- Mirror:
  Installing a full-length mirror in the training area can be useful for checking posture and body alignment during exercises. It will help you maintain proper technique and avoid injury.

- Music and atmosphere:
  Create a pleasant feeling in the practice environment. Choose relaxing or motivating music to help you focus and find the right atmosphere during practice. You can also add elements such as plants, scented candles, or soothing colors to create an environment conducive to your workout experience.

- Organization and practicality:
  Keep all the tools and equipment you need for wall Pilates practice close at hand. Make sure you have space to neatly and accessibly store mats, elastic bands, Pilates

balls, and other accessories. This will allow you to start your practice without wasting time searching for what you need.

Preparing a comfortable and functional workout environment in your home for wall Pilates will help you create a consistent routine and get the most out of your workouts. Always remember to adapt the environment according to your personal preferences and needs, creating a space that makes you feel comfortable and motivated to work out.

# Proper Posture and Breathing

When practicing Pilates on a wall, correct posture and mindful breathing are essential to get the maximum benefits from the exercises and to prevent injury.

Good posture is essential for optimal results during wall Pilates exercises. Maintaining an aligned and balanced posture during your workout will allow you to engage your muscles effectively and prevent undue stress on certain body parts. Here are some key points to keep in mind for proper posture during Pilates on the wall:

- Spinal alignment:
  Keep your spine naturally aligned, avoiding excessive bending or sagging. Imagine you have a wire lifting you from the top of your head, lengthening your spine and aligning your neck, shoulders, and pelvis.

- Active core:
  Activate the core muscles—i.e., the deep abdominals and back muscles—to support the spine and maintain a stable posture. Involve the pelvic floor muscles for additional support.

- Relaxed shoulders:
  Keep your shoulders relaxed and away from your ears. Avoid raising your shoulders or rolling them forward during exercises. Keep the shoulder blades down and slightly retracted toward the spine.

- Alignment of knees and ankles:
  Make sure your knees are aligned with your ankles and do not lean forward or backward. Keep your knees soft and slightly flexed, avoiding locking them.

Conscious breathing is a key element when performing Pilates wall exercises. Proper breathing provides oxygen to the muscles, stabilizes the core, and promotes relaxation and mental focus. Here are some tips for proper breathing during Pilates on the wall:

- Utilize diaphragmatic breathing:
  Breathe deeply and expand your diaphragm during inhalation. Imagine having your belly expand naturally during inhalation as your ribs expand laterally. During exhalation, release the air in a controlled and complete manner.

- Coordinate breathing with movement:
  Try to coordinate your breathing with the movements of the exercises. In general, inhalation occurs during preparation or relaxation, while exhalation occurs during the performance of the more challenging exercises. However, it is important to adapt breathing according to individual exercises and specific instructions.

- Practice steady, regular breathing:
  Maintain steady, regular breathing throughout the workout. Avoid holding your breath or shallow breathing. Conscious breathing promotes oxygen flow and helps maintain proper core activation.

Take the time to focus on correct posture and mindful breathing during each Pilates wall exercise. Remember that posture and breathing are key elements in getting the most benefit from this practice. Always follow the instructions and postural corrections provided by qualified instructors or reference resources to ensure that you perform the exercises correctly and safely.

With correct posture and mindful breathing, you will be able to take full advantage of the benefits of Pilates on a wall, improving strength, flexibility, and body awareness.

# Guidelines and Suggestions

Before beginning a Pilates on wall session, it is important to prepare the body through proper warm-up and preliminary muscle strengthening. This sub-chapter will provide useful guidelines to properly prepare you for Pilates on wall training.

- Heating:
  Before beginning any type of workout, it is essential to warm up the body to increase blood circulation and muscle temperature. You can perform a general warm-up that involves all major muscle groups, such as a short walk or a series of light cardio exercises such as jumping jacks. Alternatively, you can choose to perform specific exercises that involve the parts of the body that will be most stressed during wall Pilates, such as arm and leg movements.

- Stretching:
  After the warm-up, it is important to spend time stretching to lengthen and prepare your muscles for the workout. Focus on stretches that involve the major muscle groups that will be stressed during wall Pilates, such as the legs, back, and shoulders. Hold each stretch for at least 15 to 30 seconds, breathing deeply and relaxing the muscles as you stretch.

- Preliminary muscle strengthening:
  Before moving on to the more challenging wall Pilates exercises, it is advisable to spend time on preliminary muscle strengthening. Focus on exercises that involve the major muscle groups of the core, legs, and arms. You can perform exercises such as planks, squats, lunges, push-ups, and side planks to prepare the body for the strength and stability work required by Pilates on the wall. Start with low repetitions and sets, focusing on proper technique and execution of the exercises.

- Listening to your body:
  During warm-up and preliminary muscle strengthening, it is important to listen to your body and respect its limits. Do not force the exercises and avoid exceeding your comfort level. If you experience pain or discomfort, stop and consult a fitness professional or qualified Pilates instructor for personalized advice and guidance.

Properly preparing your body through warming up, stretching, and preliminary muscle strengthening will help you avoid injury and gain maximum benefits from Pilates on a wall training. Remember to spend time on this preparation phase before beginning the more challenging exercises.

# STRETCHING FOCUS

## WALL ROLL DOWN

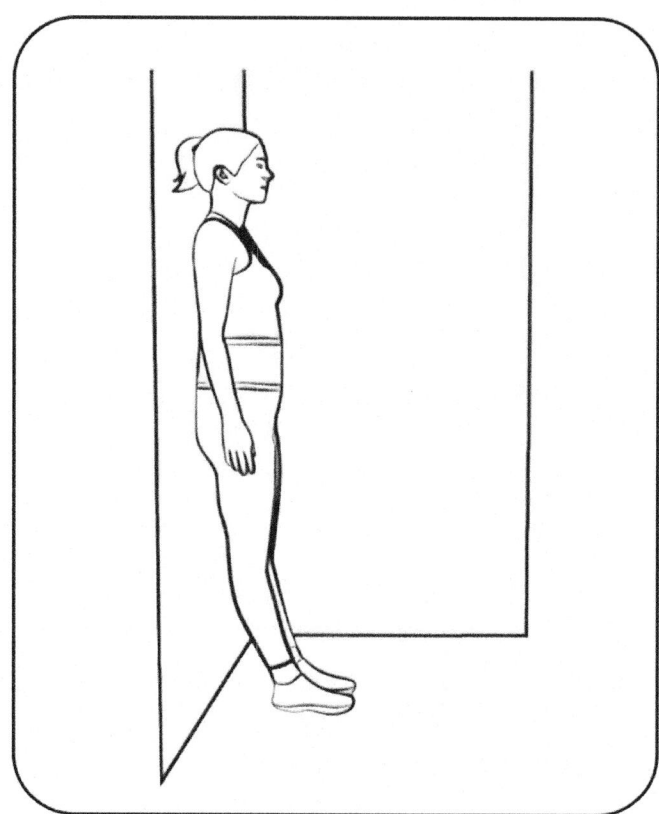 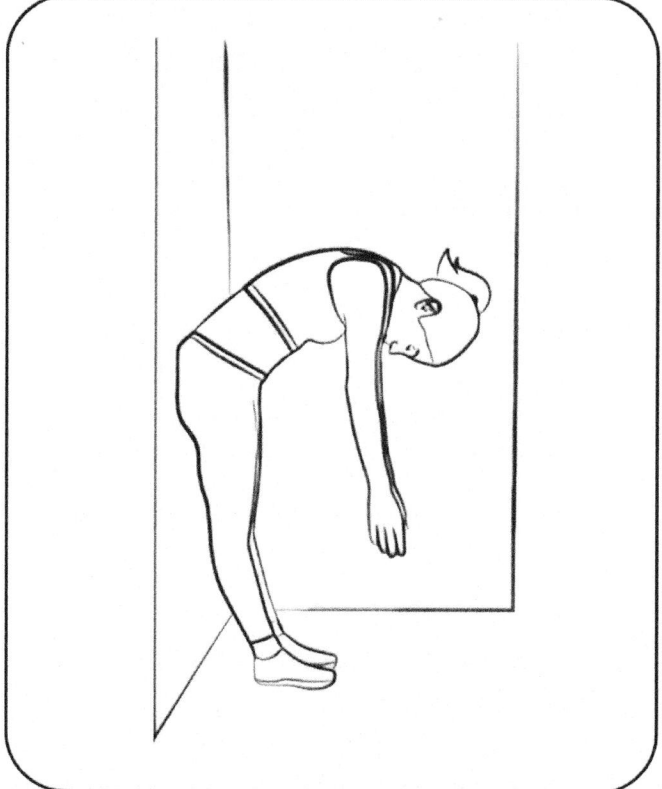

### Description

The Wall Roll Down is a Pilates exercise that aims to improve flexibility of the spine and strengthen the abdominal muscles. This position is performed with the back against the wall, providing support and stability during the movement.

10

**Execution**:
- Start standing with your back against the wall, your heels about six to eight inches away from the base of the wall, and your feet parallel and shoulder-width apart.
- Extend your arms forward at shoulder level and bend forward, trying to go to the floor with your hands.
- Upon reaching the maximum bending point, slowly begin to rise again, returning to the starting position.

**Breathing**:
- As you descend, exhale deeply to facilitate stretching of the spine and actively engage the abdominal muscles.
- As you inhale, begin to rise while maintaining control of the movement and lengthening the spine.

**Benefits**:
- Improves flexibility and mobility of the spine.
- Strengthens abdominal, lumbar, and paravertebral muscles.
- Promotes better awareness of movement and posture.

**Recommendations**:
- Keep the movement smooth and controlled, avoiding jerks or sudden movements.
- While performing, focus on breathing, synchronizing each movement with the action of the breath.
- If you have back or spine problems, consult a fitness professional or therapist before performing this exercise.

**Variants**:
- For a more advanced variation, perform the Wall Roll Down while holding your arms raised above your head, working on shoulder and arm flexibility.

# WALL ANGEL

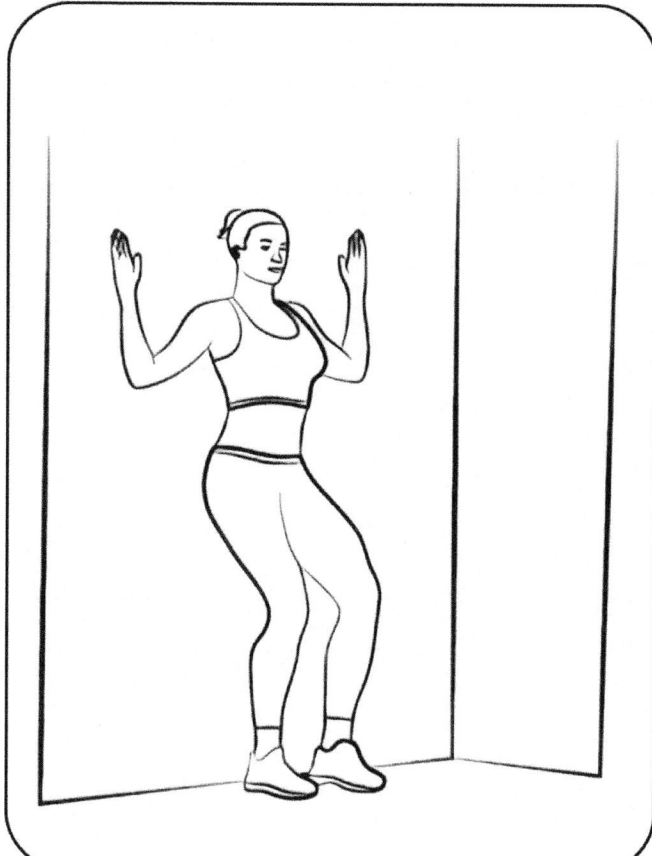 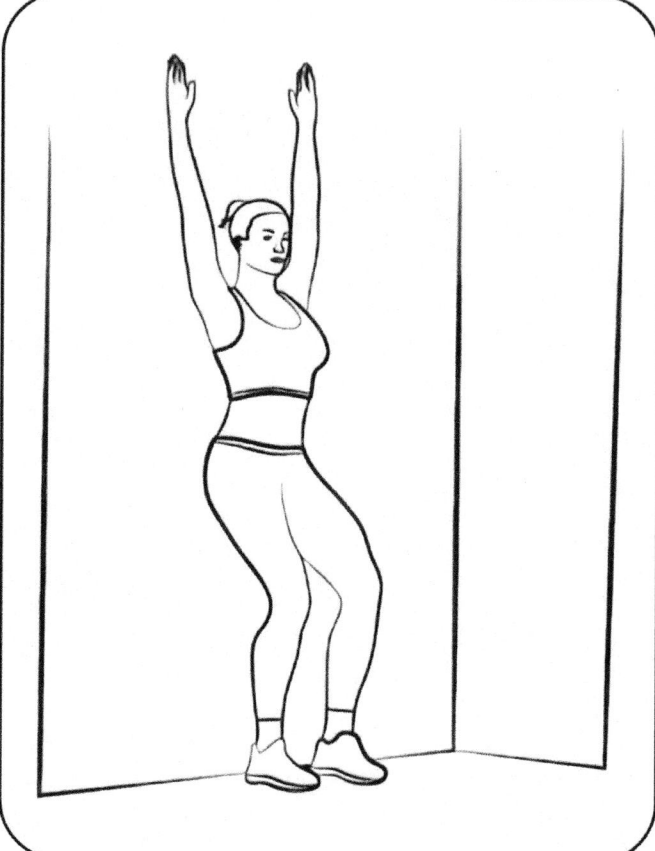

A Wall Angel is a Pilates exercise that works on shoulder mobility and stability. This position engages the shoulder and shoulder blade muscles, helping to improve posture and prevent tension in the neck and shoulder area.

**Execution**:
- Stand against the wall with your back, buttocks, and head in contact with the surface.
- Keep elbows bent at 90 degrees and arms at right angles to the body.
- Slowly, move your arms upward along the wall, gently pushing your arms up above your head.
- Make sure your elbows and wrists always maintain contact with the wall as you move your arms upward.

**Breathing**:
- Inhaling, prepare for movement.
- Exhaling, perform the upward arm movement.

**Benefits**:
- Improves mobility and flexibility of the shoulders.
- Strengthens the muscles of the scapulae and deltoids.
- Promotes correct posture and reduces tension in the neck and shoulder area.

**Recommendations**:
- Keep your back and head against the wall throughout the exercise.
- Control the movement of the arms so as to avoid overstretching the shoulders.
- If you have back or shoulder problems, consult a fitness professional or therapist before performing this exercise.

**Variants**:
- For a more intense variation, you can hold your arms outstretched during the upward movement.
- For an easier variation, you can reduce the range of motion by keeping your elbows lower than your shoulders.

# WALL SPINE STRETCH

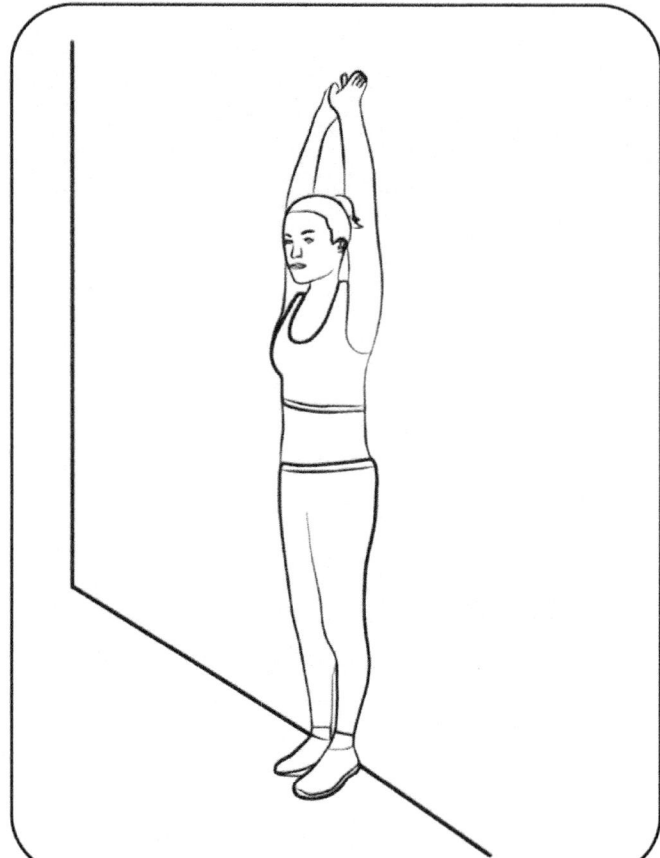 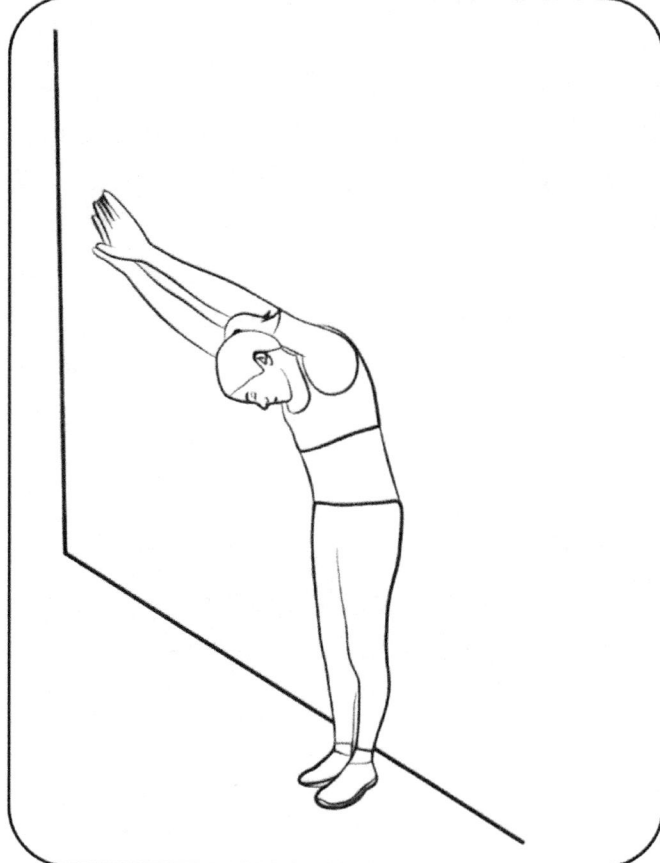

Wall Spine Stretch is a Pilates exercise that aims to improve spinal flexibility and relax tension in the upper body. By using the wall support, this exercise allows you to perform the spine stretching movement with greater precision and control.

**Execution:**
- Stand upright, with your back straight and pelvis aligned.
- Lean the back of the head against the wall, maintaining a slight curve in the lower back.
- Bring your arms above your head, palms facing the ceiling.
- Inhaling, stretch your arms upward, trying to extend your spine and lengthen your upper body.
- Exhaling, lean forward, keeping your back straight and extended.
- Repeat the movement for a few repetitions, trying to create a deep stretch in the upper back.

**Breathing:**
- Inhaling, prepare for the upward stretching movement.
- Exhaling, lean forward by lengthening the spine.

**Benefits:**
- Promotes relaxation of tension in the upper back and shoulders.
- Improves flexibility of the spine and thoracic area.
- Helps improve posture and body awareness.

**Recommendations:**
- Maintain a slight curve in the lower back while performing to avoid excessive arching of the back.
- Focus on lengthening the spine and arms as you perform the movement.
- If you have back or shoulder problems, consult a fitness professional or therapist before performing this exercise.

**Variants:**
- For a more intense variation, you can perform the Wall Spine Stretch with your arms slightly further away from the wall, increasing the lengthening of the spine and arms.
- For an easier variation, you can perform the movement only by extending your arms upward, without leaning forward.

# WALL PIKE STRETCH

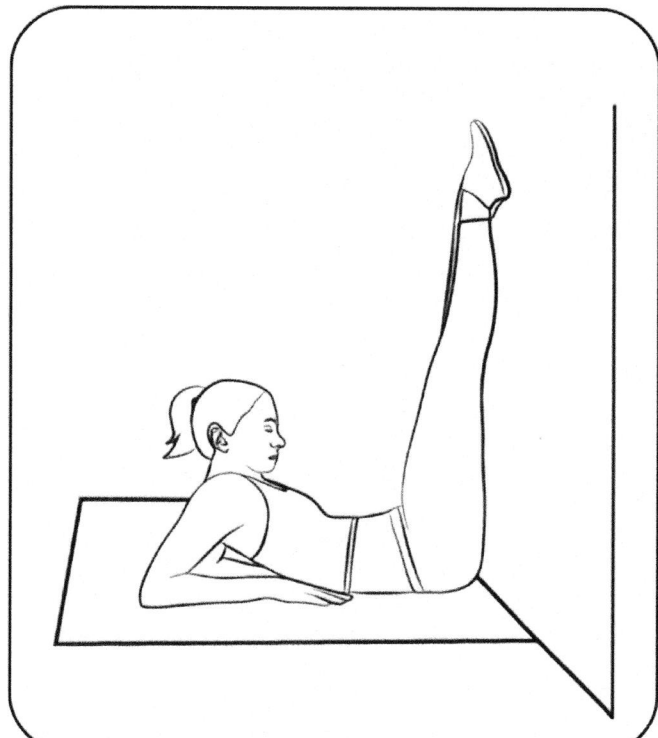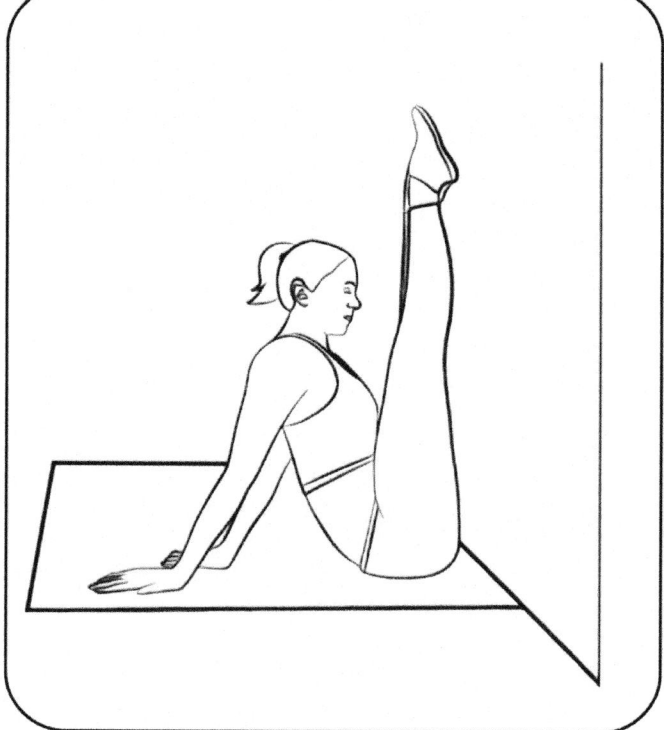

Wall Pike Stretch is an advanced Pilates exercise that aims to improve flexibility and strengthen the abdominals. Using wall support, this exercise allows you to perform an inverted V-like position, engaging different muscle groups in the back of the body.

16

**Execution:**
- Position yourself on the floor with your upper body raised on your elbows and your glutes against the wall.
- Lift both legs and place your heels against the wall, extending your legs upward and forming a right angle with your body.
- Slowly lift your torso off the floor, keeping your legs extended toward the ceiling and bending your upper body toward your legs.
- Try to bring your toes toward the ceiling as much as possible while creating a V-shaped position.
- Hold this position for a few seconds, then slowly return to the starting position.

**Breathing:**
- Breathing in, prepare for the leg and pelvis lifting movement.
- On exhaling, try to maintain the inverted V position and stretch the body.

**Benefits:**
- Improves flexibility of ischiocrucials and legs.
- Strengthens the abdominals and core stabilizing muscles.
- Promotes body coordination and balance.

**Recommendations:**
- Keep your neck and shoulders relaxed while performing the exercise.
- Avoid holding your breath; breathe in a controlled manner during movement.
- If you have back or leg problems, consult a fitness professional or therapist before performing this exercise.

**Variants:**
- For an easier variation, you can bend your knees slightly during the inverted V movement.

# WALL CHEST OPENER

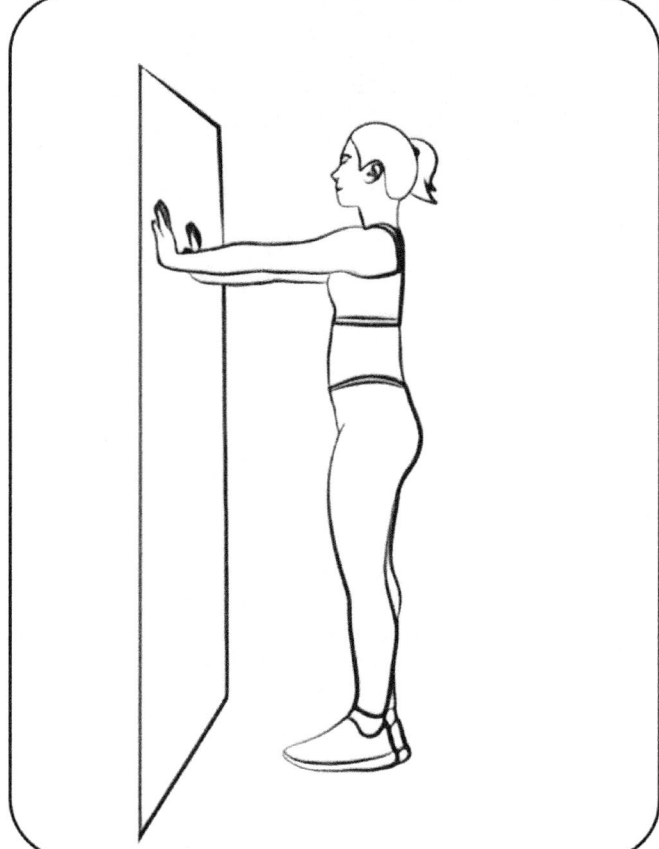 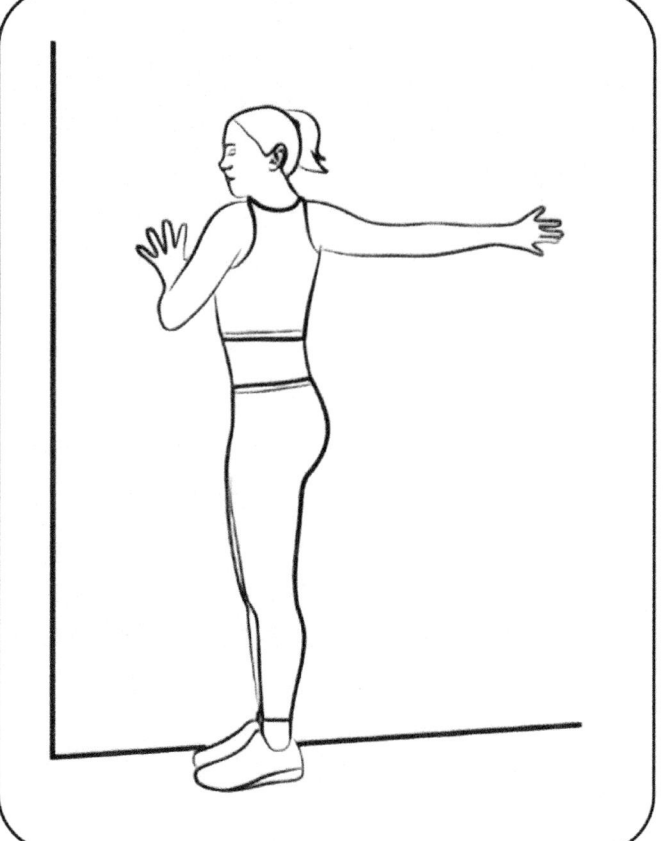

Description

Wall Chest Opener is a Pilates exercise that aims to open and lengthen the chest and shoulder muscles. Using wall support, this exercise allows you to improve flexibility and mobility of the upper body.

**Execution:**
- Stand facing the wall, with your feet slightly apart and your hands resting against the wall surface at the same height as your shoulders.
- Twist your body to the right, leaving your left arm behind you until you feel a stretch in your shoulder and chest.
- Hold this position for a few seconds.
- Slowly return to the starting position, releasing pressure on the wall.

**Breathing:**
- Inhaling, prepare for chest and arm stretching against the wall.
- Exhaling, hold the stretching position and release tension.

**Benefits:**
- Improves flexibility and mobility of the chest and shoulders.
- Relieves muscle tension in the upper body.
- Promotes correct and open posture of the chest.

**Recommendations:**
- Avoid excessive pushing against the wall; keep the stretch controlled and comfortable.
- Keep your neck and shoulders relaxed while performing the exercise.
- If you have shoulder or chest problems, consult a fitness professional or therapist before performing this exercise.

**Variants:**
- For an easier variation, you can perform the exercise with your hands placed at a lower height on the wall, thus reducing the intensity of the stretch.

# WALL SHOULDER STRETCH

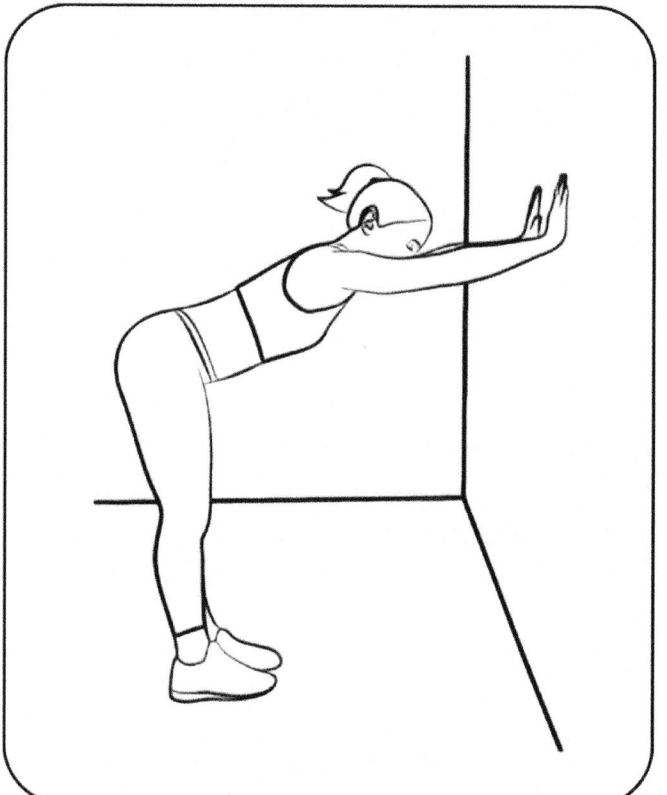 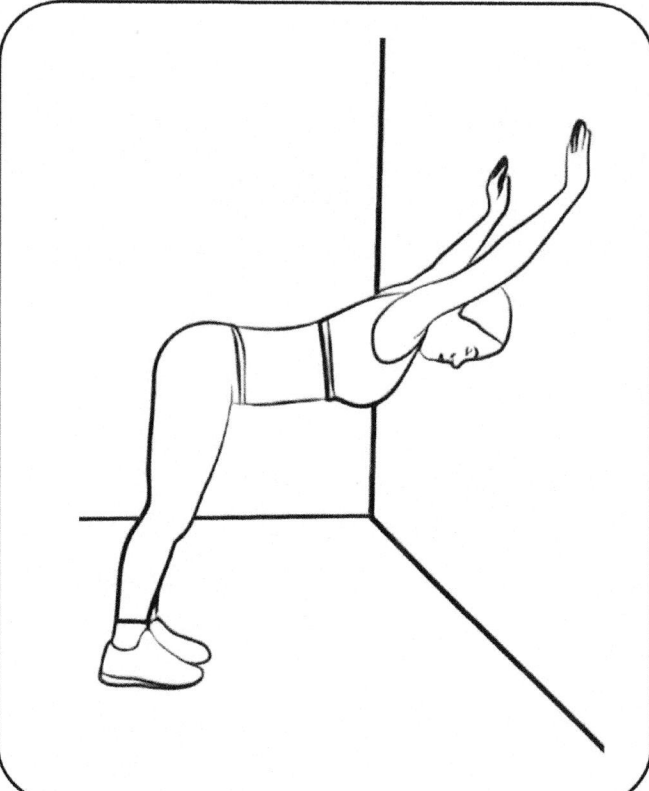

## Description

*The Wall Shoulder Stretch is a stretching and flexibility exercise ideal for relaxing and stretching the muscles of the shoulders, chest, and back. This movement promotes improved shoulder mobility and upper body flexibility, helping to prevent muscle tension and stiffness.*

**Execution:**
- Stand facing the wall with feet aligned at shoulder height and legs slightly bent.
- Lean forward from the waist, bringing the torso to an angle of about 90 degrees to the legs. Your arms should be fully extended and resting against the wall at a height slightly above your shoulders.
- Move your feet away from the wall a few inches so as to create a slight tension in your upper body.
- Hold the stretching position for 20–30 seconds, breathing deeply and relaxed.

**Breathing:**
- Inhaling deeply, prepare for the exercise, bringing attention to your posture and correct execution.
- Exhaling slowly, bend your torso forward and stretch your arms over the wall, feeling the stretching sensation in your upper body.

**Benefits:**
- Relaxes and stretches the muscles of the shoulders, chest, and back.
- Promotes improved mobility and flexibility of shoulder joints, helping to prevent pain and muscle tension caused by poor posture or daily activities.
- Helps relax tension in the shoulder and neck area, relieving symptoms of stress and improving overall well-being.

**Recommendations:**
- Be sure to maintain proper posture while performing the exercise, keeping your torso well aligned with your legs.
- Do not force the stretch and avoid overextending the arms while performing it. The stretch should be gentle and comfortable.

**Variants:**
- To increase the intensity of the stretch, you can vary the height of your arms on the wall. By raising your arms, you're going to stimulate different muscles in your shoulders and chest.
- You can also perform the Wall Shoulder Stretch with one knee bent and the other extended to accentuate the stretch in the shoulder and chest area.

# WALL SIDE BEND

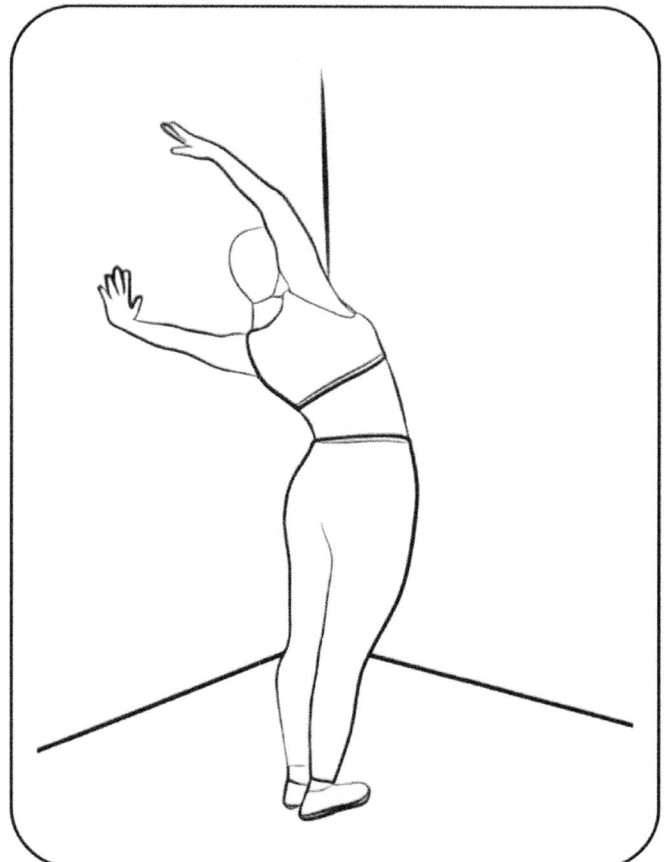 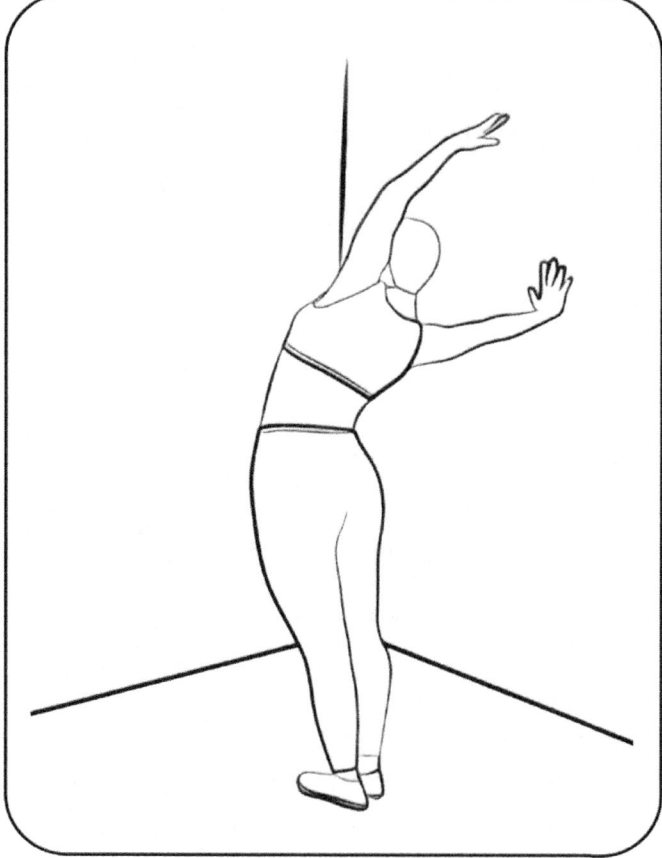

The Wall Side Bend is a lateral stretching exercise that involves the oblique and side muscles of the body. This movement helps to improve flexibility and mobility of the spine, promoting reduction of tension in the shoulder and hip areas.

**Execution:**
- Stand sideways to the wall, with your left side facing the wall. Your legs should be slightly apart and your feet aligned with your shoulders.
- Raise your right arm above your head, extending it fully so that it is parallel to the wall. The palm of the hand should be facing the ceiling.
- Bring the left arm against the wall, resting the forearm on the vertical surface and aligning the elbow with the shoulder.
- From this position, tilt your torso sideways toward the wall, pushing your left hip to the left and keeping your right arm outstretched above your head. The goal is to create a lateral curve in the spine and feel a stretch along the right side of the body.
- Hold the stretch position for 20–30 seconds, breathing deeply and regularly.
- Slowly return to the starting position and then repeat the movement on the opposite side.

**Breathing:**
- Inhaling deeply, prepare for the exercise, bringing attention to your posture and correct execution.
- Exhaling slowly, tilt your torso sideways toward the wall, feeling the stretch along the side of your body.
- Maintain regular and continuous breathing throughout the exercise.

**Benefits:**
- Improves flexibility and mobility of the spine, helping to prevent tension and stiffness in the hip and shoulder area.
- Stimulates the oblique muscles, which are responsible for lateral movement of the trunk, helping to strengthen and tone the side of the body.
- Promotes better postural alignment, reducing compression on the spine and promoting better overall posture.

**Recommendations:**
- Be sure to maintain proper posture while performing the exercise, avoiding excessive bending of the back or pushing the hips forward.
- Do not force the stretch and always keep control of the movements to avoid injury or discomfort.

**Variants:**
- To increase the intensity of the stretch, you can push the hip even more toward the wall, trying to create a more pronounced curve in the spine.

## KNEE TO CHEST

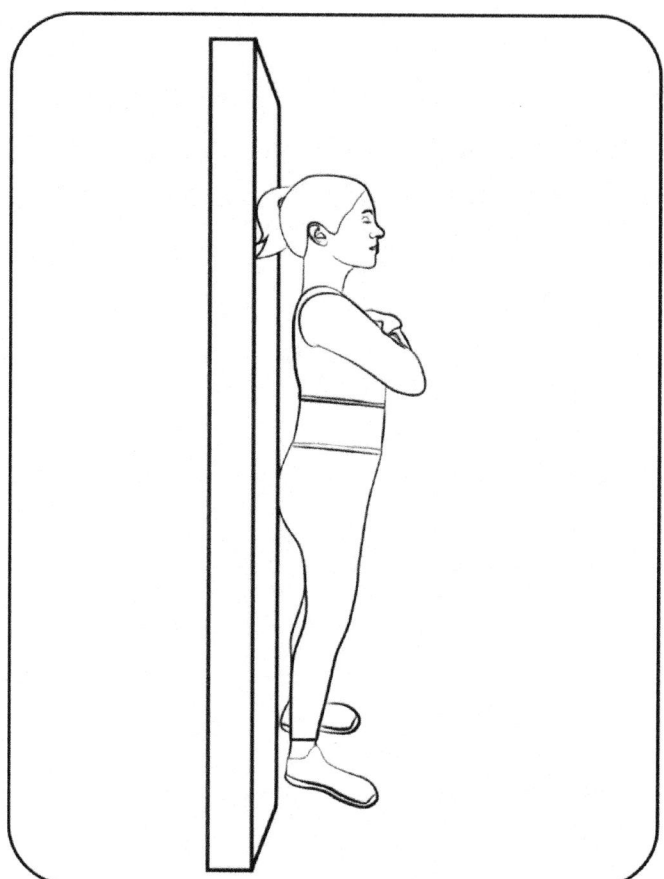 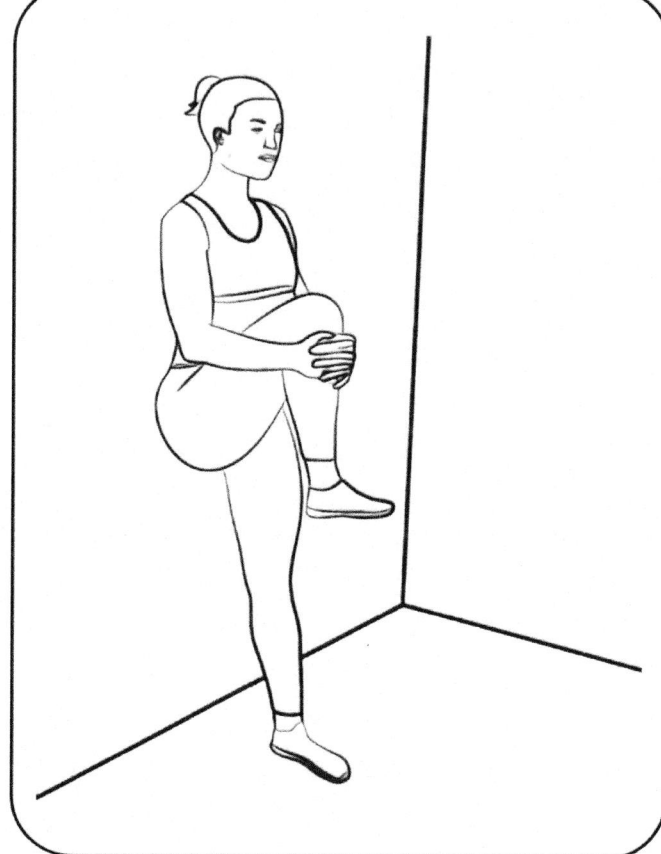

### Description

*Knee to Chest is a simple stretching exercise that helps relieve tension and pain in the lower back by promoting flexibility of the hip flexors and improving mobility of the hip and knee joints.*

24

**Execution:**
- Position yourself with your back against the wall and your feet placed about two feet away from the wall.
- Lift your right foot off the floor and bring your knee toward your chest. You can help by wrapping your hands around the front of the knee and applying gentle upward pressure to increase the stretch.
- Hold the position for about 30 seconds, breathing deeply and relaxing the muscles.
- Slowly release the knee and repeat the exercise with the left leg.

**Breathing:**
- Inhaling, prepare for the exercise and bring the knee toward the chest.
- As you exhale, relax the muscles and deepen the stretch, keeping your breathing regular and fluid.

**Benefits:**
- Relieves hip flexor stiffness, which can be caused by long hours of sitting or poor posture.
- Promotes relaxation of lower back muscles, helping to reduce pain and tension in the lower back.
- Improves flexibility and mobility of hip and knee joints, promoting smoother movement and greater agility in daily activities.

**Recommendations:**
- Be sure to perform the exercise calmly and carefully, avoiding sudden or forced movements.
- Do not overstretch or pull the knee excessively toward the chest. Always maintain a feeling of comfort and never pain.

**Variants:**
- You can perform this exercise in a sitting position in a chair or on an elevated surface if standing is too challenging.

# CORE FOCUS

## WALL TEASER

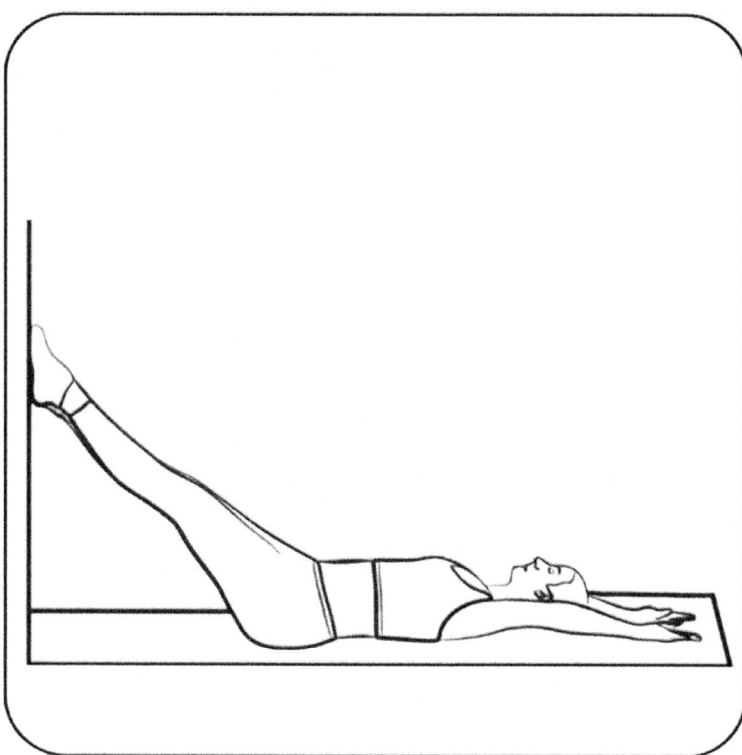 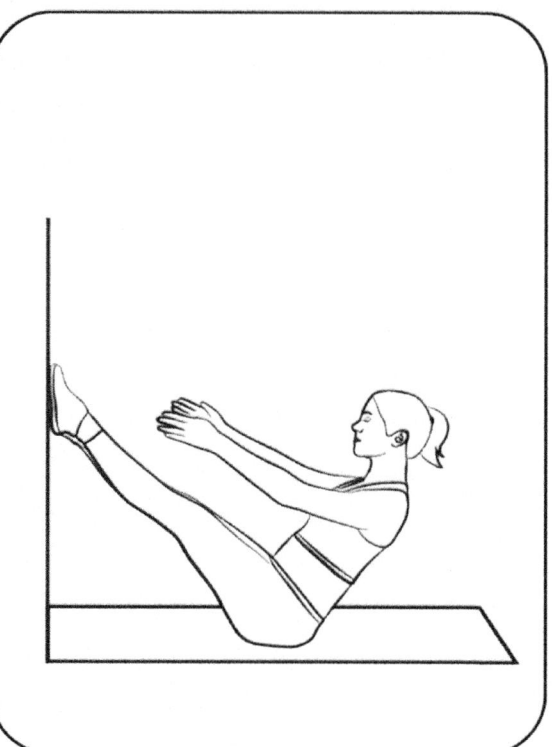

### Description

Wall Teaser is an advanced Pilates exercise involving the core, upper and lower abdominals, and leg muscles. This position requires strength, balance, and body control and is an advanced variation of the traditional Teaser, taking advantage of the wall support to provide stability while performing.

**Execution:**
- Lie on the floor, with your back straight and your legs stretched out in front of you.
- Lean your feet up against the wall with your arms stretched forward.
- Start by lifting your torso off the floor, keeping your legs outstretched and forming a "V" with your body.
- Hold the position for a few seconds, trying to maintain balance and body alignment.
- Slowly release the position and return to the starting position.

**Breathing:**
- Inhaling, prepare for the leg and torso lifting movement.
- As you exhale, simultaneously raise your legs and torso from the sitting position.
- Inhaling again, hold the raised position for a few seconds.
- Exhaling, slowly release the position and return to the floor.

**Benefits:**
- Strengthens upper and lower abdominals.
- Promotes movement control and balance.

**Recommendations:**
- Before you try the Wall Teaser, make sure you have good core strength.
- Keep your back straight and aligned while performing the exercise to avoid excessive stress on the lower back.

**Variants:**
- For a more intense variation, you can perform the Wall Teaser without the wall support.
- For an easier variation, you can perform the Wall Teaser with your knees bent, reducing the range of motion. As you become more comfortable, you can gradually extend your legs.

# WALL SIDE PLANK

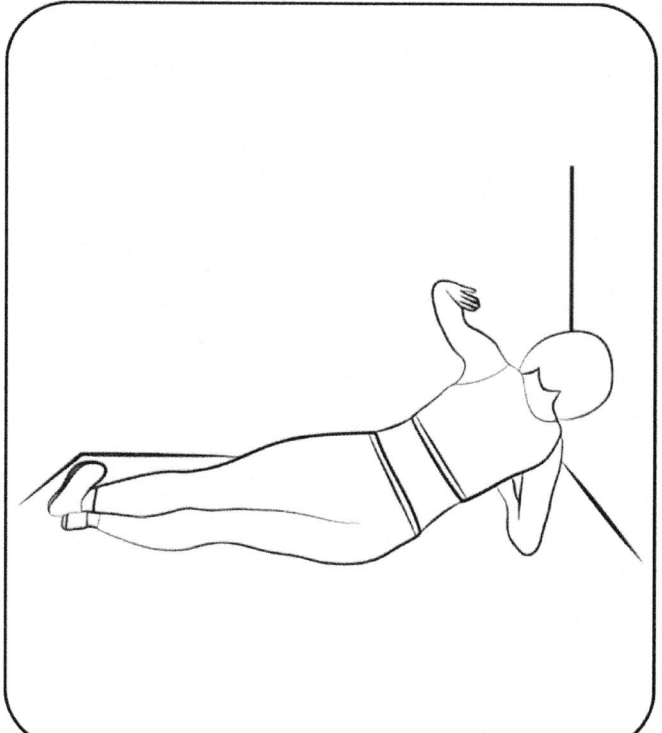 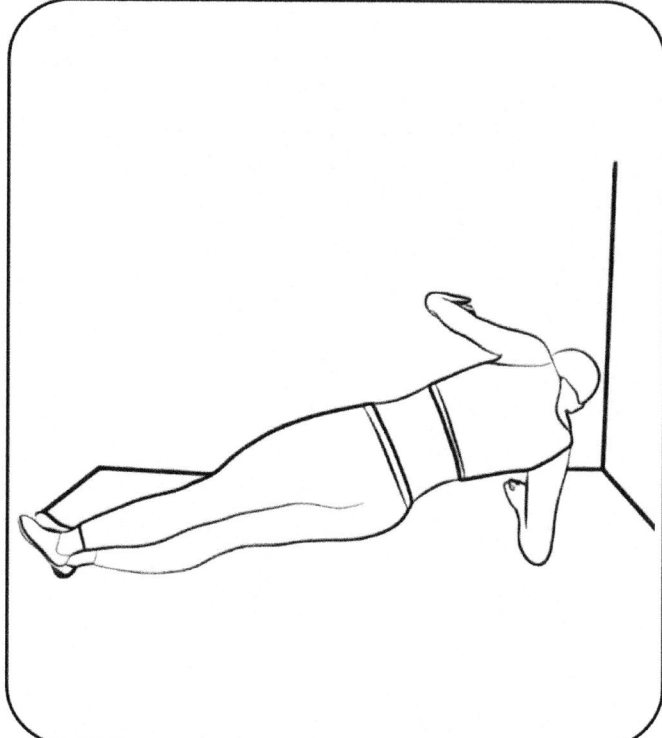

Wall Side Plank is an advanced Pilates exercise that aims to strengthen the oblique abdominals and trunk stabilizers. Using wall support, this exercise allows you to perform the Plank position in a controlled and precise manner, focusing on the side muscles of the body.

**Execution**:
- Position yourself sideways to the wall, lying on your right side.
- Rest your right elbow on the floor, aligning it with your shoulder.
- Rest the palm of the left hand against the wall to stabilize the body.
- Lift the pelvis off the floor, forming a straight line from foot to head.
- Contract your abs and glutes to keep your body stable in the Side Plank position.
- Hold this position for a few seconds, then switch sides and repeat on the other side.

**Breathing**:
- Inhaling, prepare for pelvic lift in the Side Plank position.
- Exhaling, contract the abdominals and buttocks to keep the position stable.

**Benefits**:
- Strengthens oblique abdominals and trunk stabilizers.
- Improves balance and lateral stability of the body.
- Promotes strengthening of back and shoulder muscles.

**Recommendations**:
- Keep the body aligned and the pelvis raised to avoid lowering the hip toward the floor.
- Keep your neck and shoulders relaxed while performing the exercise.

**Variants**:
- For a more intense variation, you can lift the top foot off the ground, creating a greater effort of balance and stability.
- For an easier variation, you can bend your lower leg slightly and rest your knee on the floor, providing more support while performing the Wall Side Plank.

# WALL BICYCLE CRUNCHES

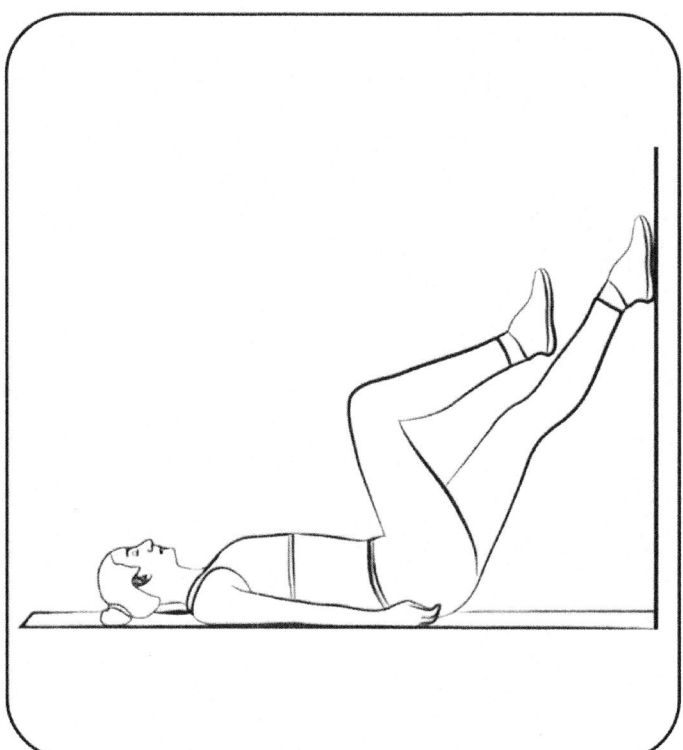 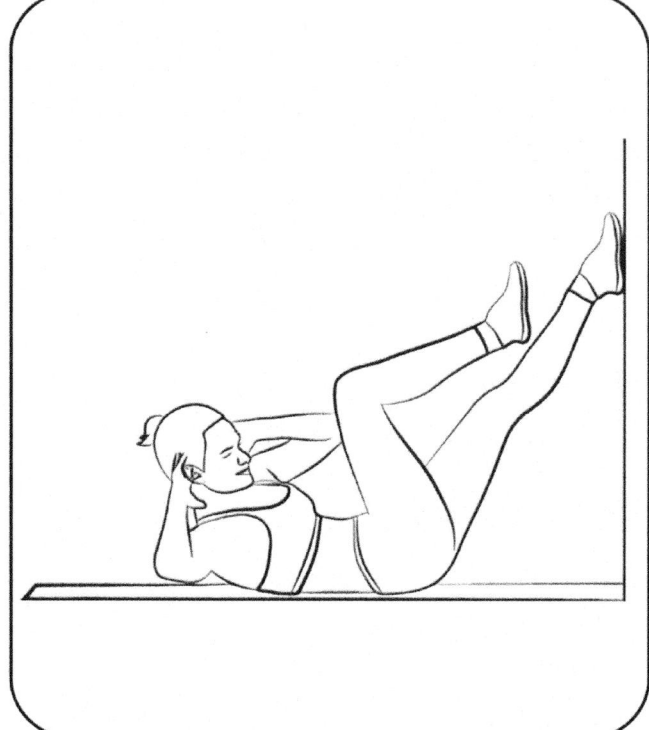

## Description

*A Wall Bicycle Crunch is an advanced Pilates exercise that involves the abdominal, oblique, and hip flexor muscles. Using the wall for support, this exercise provides stability and allows you to focus on working the abdominal muscles effectively.*

**Execution:**
- Lie on the floor, with your back firmly supported and your legs stretched upward against the wall.
- Place your hands behind your head, with your elbows pointing outward.
- Lift the torso slightly, keeping the neck relaxed and looking upward.
- Bring your right knee toward your chest as you extend your left leg upward against the wall.
- At the same time, bring the left elbow toward the right knee, performing a torso twist.
- Return to the starting position and then perform the opposite movement.

**Breathing:**
- Inhaling, prepare for movement.
- Exhaling, perform the twisting motion by bringing the right knee toward the chest and the left elbow toward the right knee.
- Inhaling, return to the starting position.
- Exhaling, perform the opposite movement.

**Benefits:**
- Strengthens and tones the abdominal, oblique and hip flexor muscles.
- Improves flexibility of the spine and lumbar region.
- Promotes core coordination and balance.

**Recommendations:**
- Maintain a constant abdominal contraction to stabilize the core during the movement.
- Avoid pulling the neck during the exercise, focusing on activating the abdominal muscles.

**Variants:**
- For a more intense variation, you can increase the number of repetitions or perform the exercise with greater speed.
- For an easier variation, you can perform the exercise by keeping your feet against the wall during the movement, thus reducing the extension of your legs.

# WALL CRUNCH

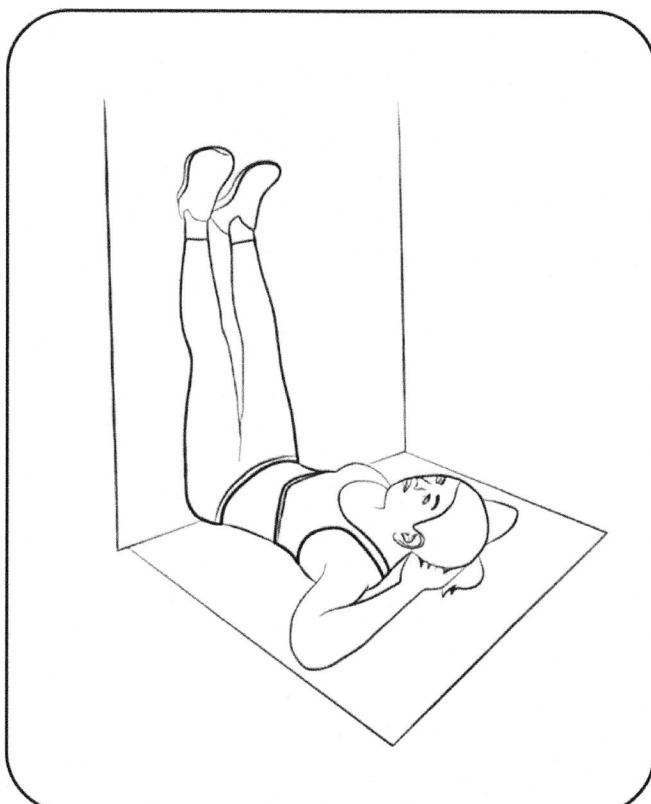 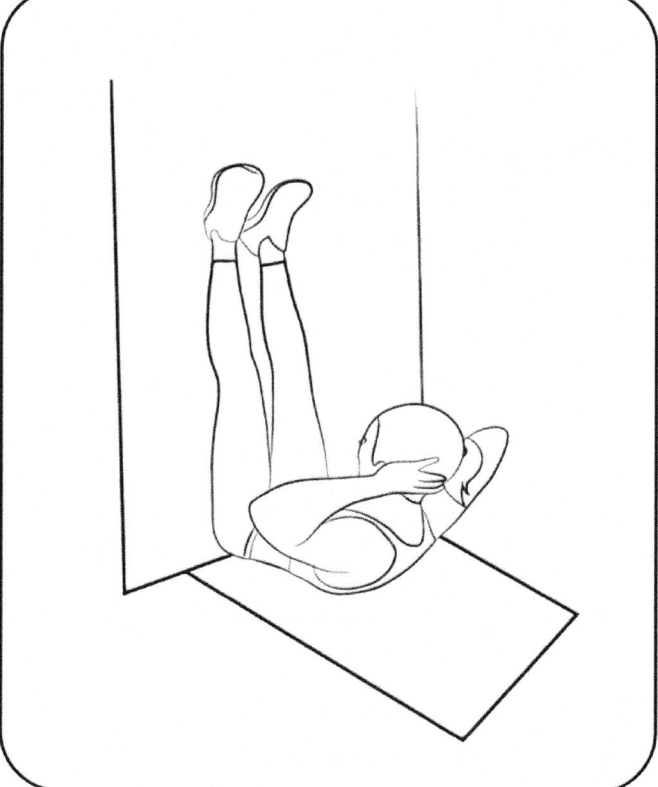

## Description

*The Wall Crunch is a wall Pilates exercise that aims to strengthen the abdominals and improve the flexibility of the spine. This exercise involves the upper and lower abdominal muscles, helping to tone the core area of the body.*

**Execution**:
- Lie on your back with your buttocks resting against the wall and your legs extended vertically along the wall. The legs should be together and the feet slightly flexed.
- Place your hands behind your head, crossing your fingers, without forcing your neck or nape up.
- Contract your abs and gently lift your torso off the floor, bringing your shoulder blades upward.
- Proceed with the movement until your abdominal muscles are fully contracted and you feel a slight flexion in your torso.
- Pause briefly in the maximum contraction position and then slowly lower your torso back to the starting position.
- Repeat the movement for the desired number of repetitions.

**Breathing**:
- Inhaling, prepare for the movement by relaxing the abdominal muscles.
- As you exhale, contract your abdominals and gently lift your torso.
- Inhaling, hold the position of maximum contraction.
- Exhaling, lower the torso, returning to the starting position.

**Benefits**:
- Strengthens the abdominals, improving trunk stability.
- Helps increase the flexibility of the spine.
- Helps develop better body awareness and alignment when performing Pilates exercises.

**Recommendations**:
- Avoid forcing the neck or nape up during the exercise, focusing on the abdominals to lift the upper body.
- Always maintain regular breathing during movement to facilitate fluidity of movement.
- Start with a limited number of repetitions and gradually increase as you gain more strength and flexibility.

**Variants**:
- To make the exercise more challenging, you can hold a small weight or Pilates ball in your hands during the movement.
- If you need an easier variation, you can reduce the range of motion by lifting your torso only slightly off the ground or keeping your feet bent on the wall while performing.

# WALL LATERAL CRUNCH

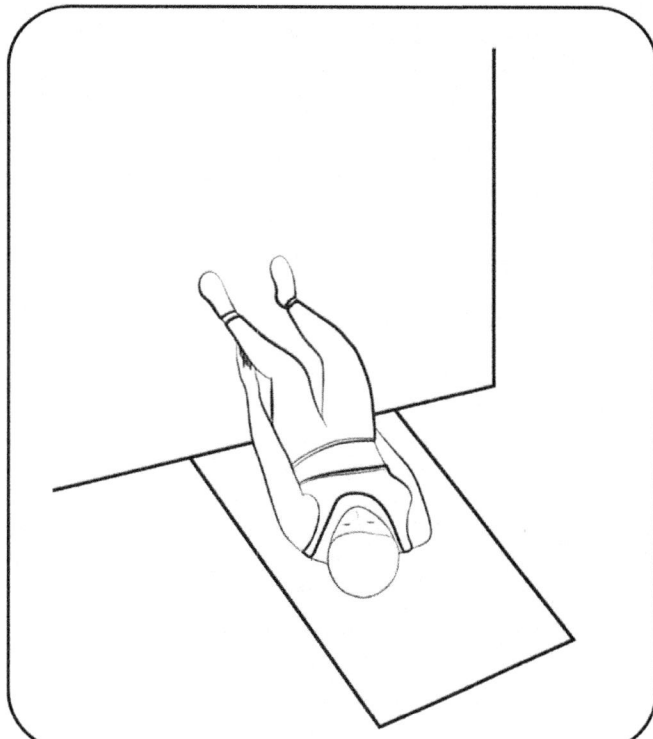 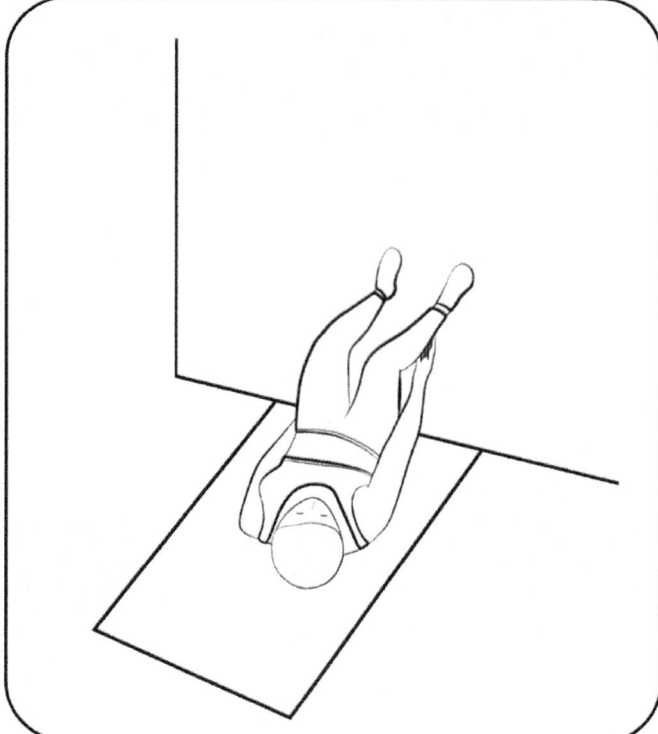

## Description

The Wall Lateral Crunch is a wall Pilates exercise that aims to strengthen the lateral abdominals, also known as the obliques. This movement involves the abdominal muscles and lateral flexion of the torso, helping to develop stability and tone in the core area of the body.

**Execution**:

- Lie on the floor with your buttocks against the wall and legs bent at 90 degrees. Your feet are against the wall, creating a right angle between your legs and the floor.
- Extend your arms sideways on the floor, aligned with your body.
- Contract your abdominals and lift your torso off the floor, directing the movement to the left. During this movement, bring your left hand toward your left foot, trying to touch it or get as close as possible.
- Pause briefly in the position of maximum contraction, feeling the work of the lateral abdominals.
- Slowly return to the starting position and repeat the movement on the right side, bringing the right hand toward the right foot.

**Breathing**:

- Inhaling, prepare for the movement by maintaining a relaxed posture.
- Exhaling, contracting the abdominals, lift the torso and direct the movement to the left or right.
- Inhaling, hold the position of maximum contraction.
- Exhaling, return to the starting position.

**Benefits**:

- Strengthens and tones the lateral abdominals, helping to develop greater trunk stability.
- Promotes lateral bending of the torso, improving flexibility of the spine.
- Stimulates oblique muscles, allowing greater control of body movement.

**Recommendations**:

- While performing the exercise, maintain correct posture, avoiding arching your back or forcing your neck up.
- Focus on the side abdominals during the movement, avoiding straining the neck or other parts of the body.

**Variants**:

- To increase the intensity of the exercise, you can hold a small weight or Pilates ball in your hands during the movement.
- If you need an easier variation, you can reduce the amplitude of the movement or rest only one hand on the floor during execution.

# WALL PLANK

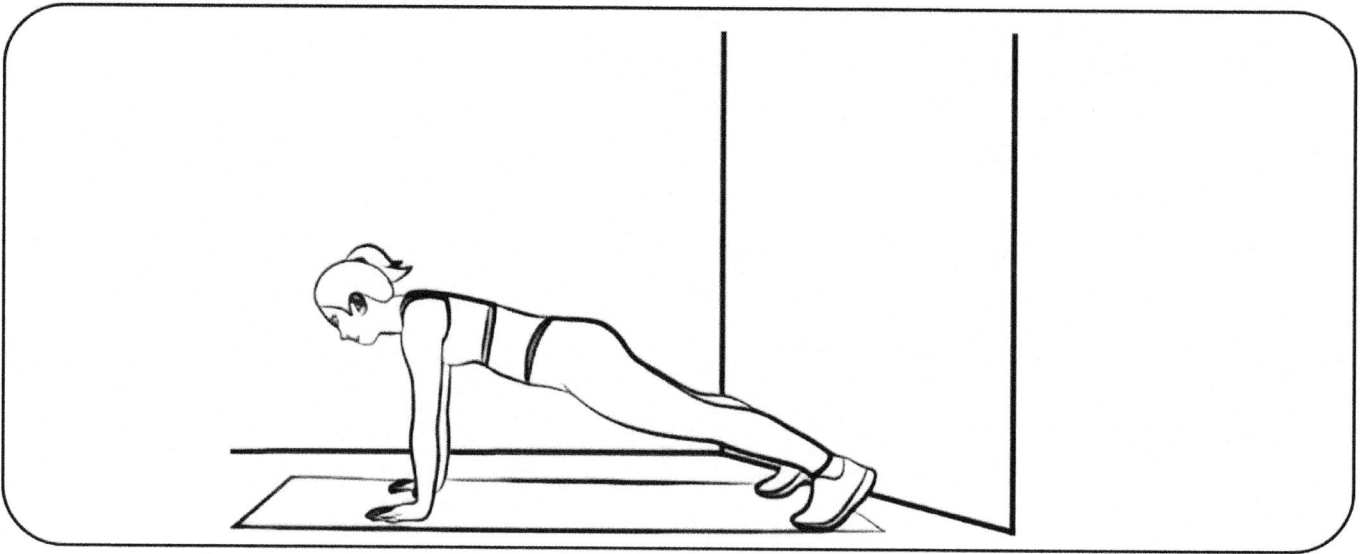

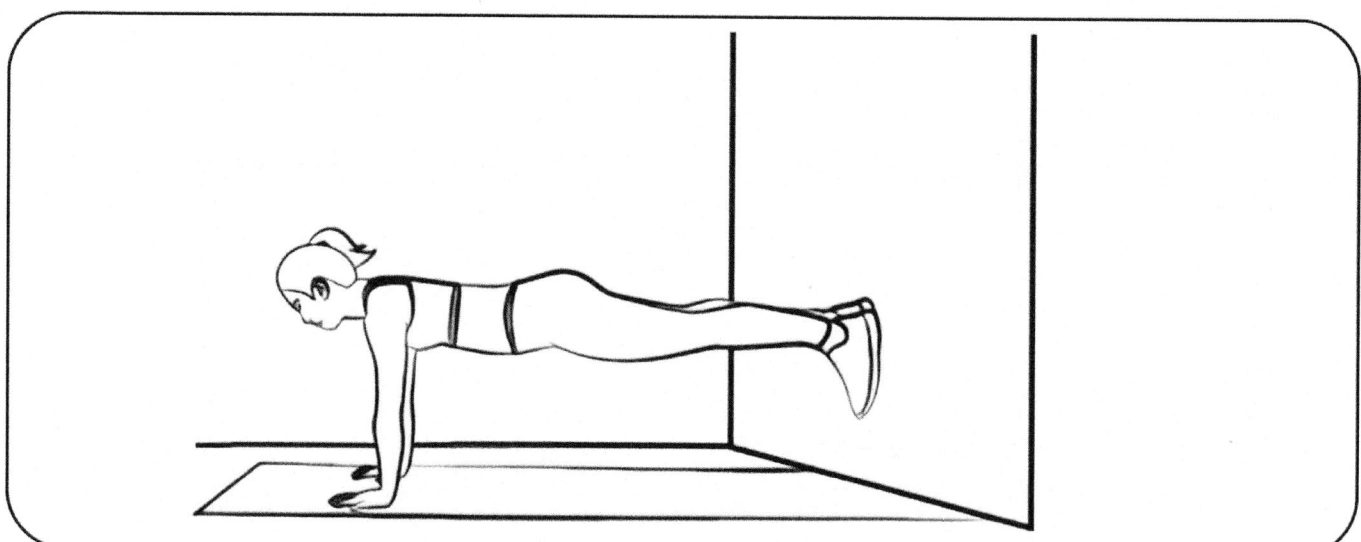

## Description

The Wall Plank is a wall-based Pilates exercise that involves several muscle groups, particularly the abdominals, arm and shoulder muscles, and leg muscles. This variation of the traditional plank is performed with both feet resting on the base of the wall, adding an element of challenge and intensity to the exercise.

**Execution:**
- Stand facing away from the wall and then get into a plank position, with your hands extended on the floor, aligned with your shoulders and palms firmly on the floor.
- The elbows should be slightly flexed and the body in a straight line from neck to heels, with the abdominals contracted.
- Once in plank position, lift both feet off the floor and start pushing against the wall.
- Gradually move the feet upward until they are aligned at shoulder height or desired level.
- Hold the position for a few seconds, keeping the body in alignment and the abdominals tightly contracted.
- Slowly come down with your feet on the floor and repeat the movement.

**Breathing:**
- Inhaling, prepare for the movement by maintaining a relaxed posture.
- Exhaling, contracting the abdominals, lift both feet, and bring them closer to the chest.
- Inhaling, hold the plank position while bringing both feet against the wall.
- Exhaling, hold the Wall Plank position.

**Benefits:**
- Strengthens and tones the abdominals, arms, and shoulders, helping to improve trunk stability.
- Involves the leg muscles, increasing the endurance and strength of this region.
- Improves coordination and body awareness.

**Recommendations:**
- Maintain correct posture, avoiding arching your back or lifting your hips while performing.
- Keep your abdominal muscles tightly contracted to support your body in plank position.

**Variants:**
- If you need an easier variation, you can perform the Wall Plank by placing your feet on the base of the wall and your hands on the floor.
- To increase the intensity, you can try lifting one leg off the wall while performing the Wall Plank or alternate between lifting legs to work asymmetrically.

# WALL PLANK PUSH

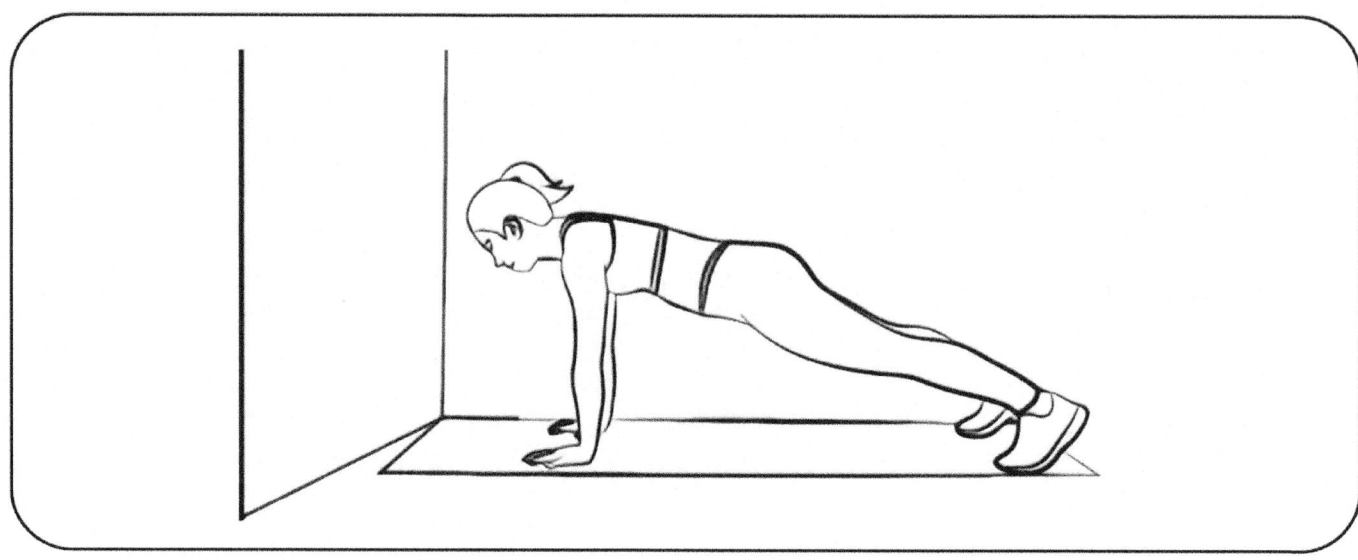

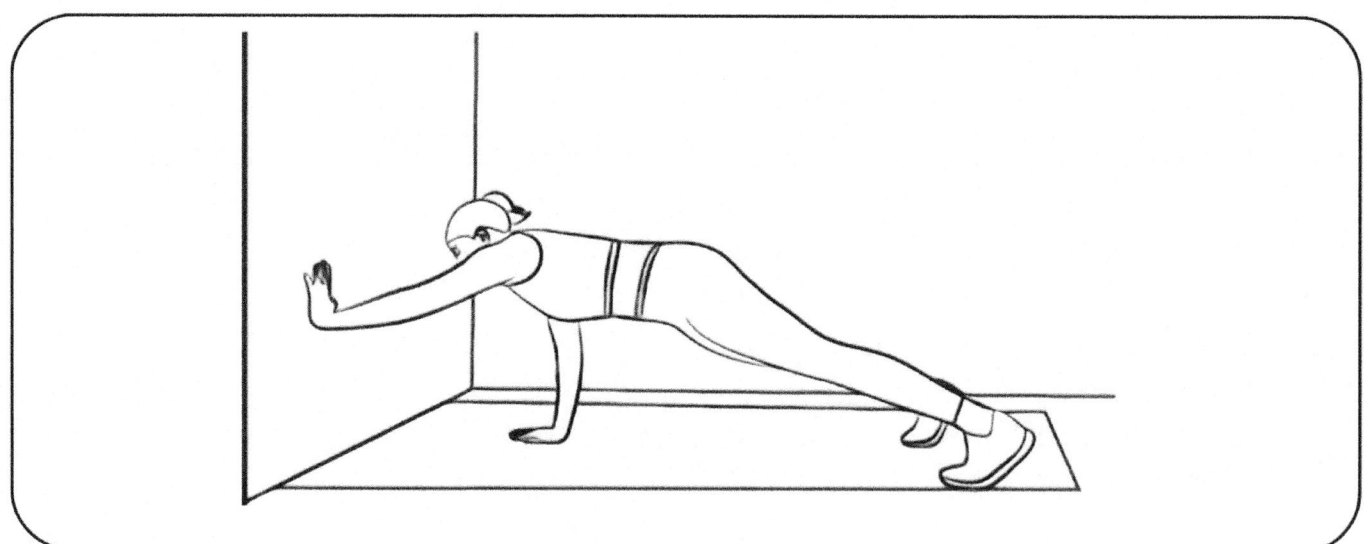

## Description

The Wall Plank Push is an advanced variation of the traditional plank that intensely engages the muscles of the arms, shoulders, and core. The exercise requires strength and control to maintain stability while extending one hand toward the wall.

**Execution:**
- Get into a plank position facing the wall, with arms fully extended and hands positioned about three feet from the wall.
- Make sure the shoulders are aligned above the wrists and the body forms a straight line from head to toe.
- Begin execution by contracting the abdominals and glutes to stabilize the body.
- Reach out one hand and place it against the wall, keeping the other hand on the ground to support the weight of the body.
- Hold the position for 10 to 15 seconds, then switch sides, extending the other hand against the wall.

**Breathing:**
- Inhaling, prepare for the exercise and stabilize the body in a plank position.
- As you exhale, extend one hand toward the wall and maintain regular breathing during the exercise.

**Benefits:**
- Strengthens the muscles of the arms and shoulders, particularly the triceps and deltoids.
- Actively involves the core muscles, helping to develop stability and strength in the abdominal region.
- Promotes improved balance and coordination, as it requires good body control while stretching one hand toward the wall.

**Recommendations:**
- Before trying the Wall Plank Push, make sure you have a good command of the traditional plank.
- Keep the spine aligned while performing, avoiding lifting the hips or dropping the pelvis.
- If you have shoulder or wrist problems, perform the exercise with caution or avoid it altogether.

**Variants:**
- To simplify the exercise, you can perform the traditional plank without extending one hand toward the wall.
- To increase the intensity, you can perform more repetitions with both hands against the wall before switching sides, or you can try holding the position for a longer period of time.

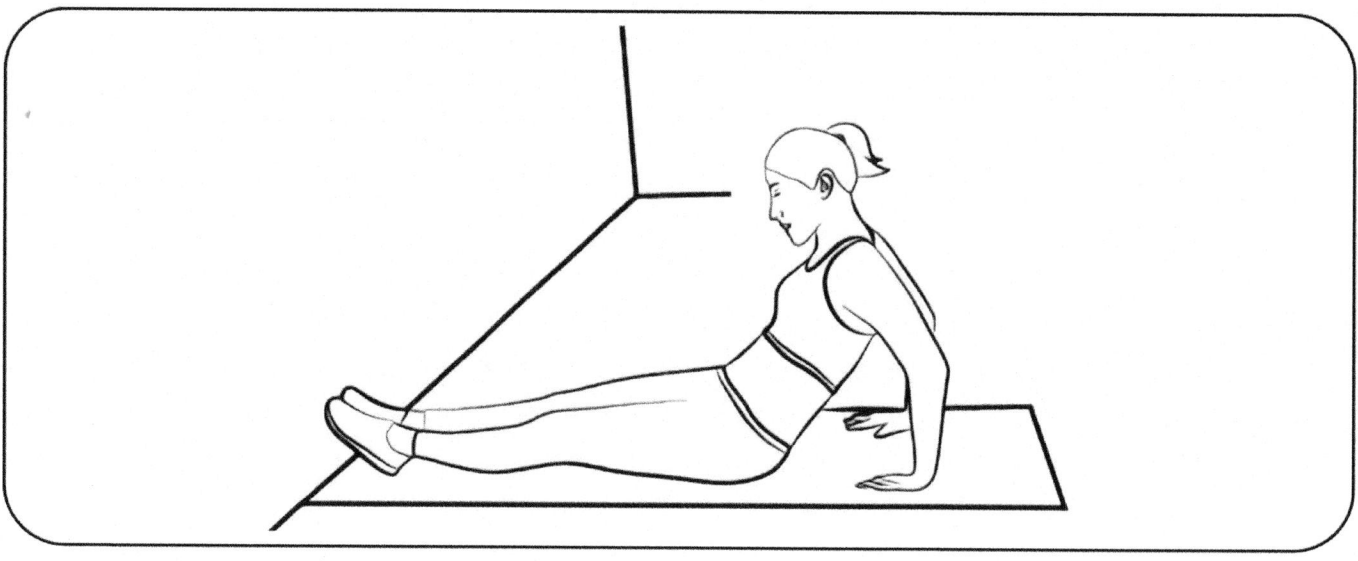

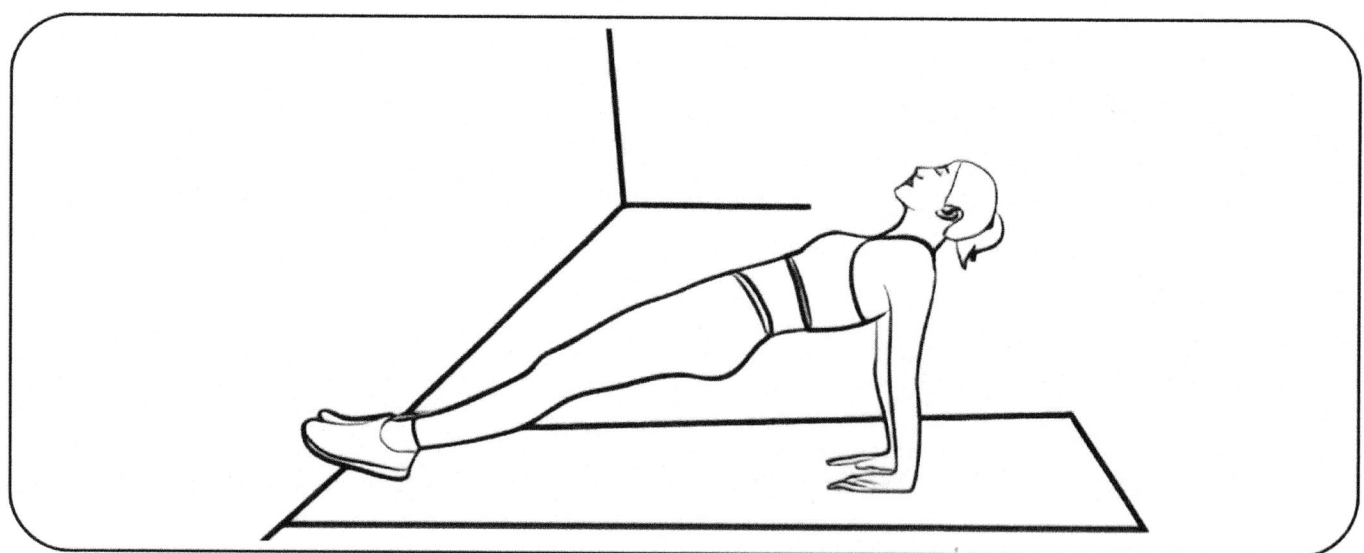

**Description**

The Wall Reverse Plank is an exercise that engages the upper body and core, helping to strengthen and tone the upper limbs, back, abs, and legs. This position requires stability and control to keep the body in a straight line.

**Execution:**
- Position yourself seated with your feet resting on the base of the wall and your hands resting behind your back, just outside your hips. Your fingers should be pointing toward your feet.
- Push through the hands and heels, lifting the pelvis upward. The body will form a straight line from the shoulders to the feet.
- Keep your neck relaxed and your gaze directed toward the ceiling to keep your spine aligned.
- Focus on contracting the buttocks and abdomen to support the weight of the body.
- Hold the position for 20–30 seconds, breathing deeply and maintaining control.

**Breathing:**
- Inhaling, prepare for the exercise and push through your hands and feet.
- As you exhale, contract your abdominals and glutes, maintaining regular, controlled breathing throughout the exercise.

**Benefits:**
- Strengthens the upper limbs, particularly the triceps and shoulder muscles.
- Helps tone core muscles, improving spinal stability and promoting correct posture.
- Stresses the muscles of the back, buttocks, and legs, helping to improve overall body strength.

**Recommendations:**
- Be sure to keep your shoulders away from your ears, avoiding loading your weight on the neck area.
- Control your breathing while performing to keep your body stable and balanced.
- If you have shoulder, wrist, or neck problems, consult a fitness professional or physical therapist before performing this exercise.

**Variants:**
- To make the exercise more challenging, you can lift one leg at a time and hold the position on your arms and one foot.
- To simplify the position, you can keep your pelvis elevated but bend your legs to 90 degrees and keep your heels on the ground, thus reducing the weight you have to support.

# FULL BODY FOCUS

## WALL PUSH-UP

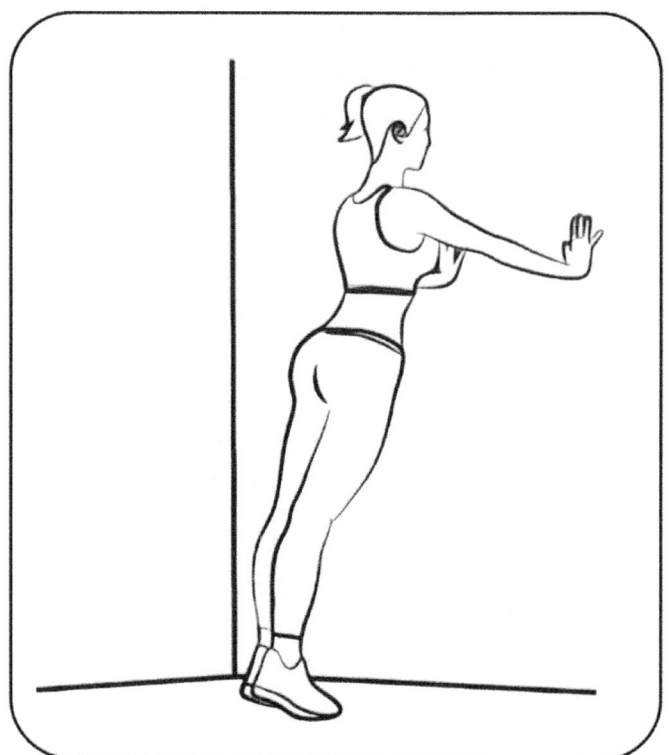 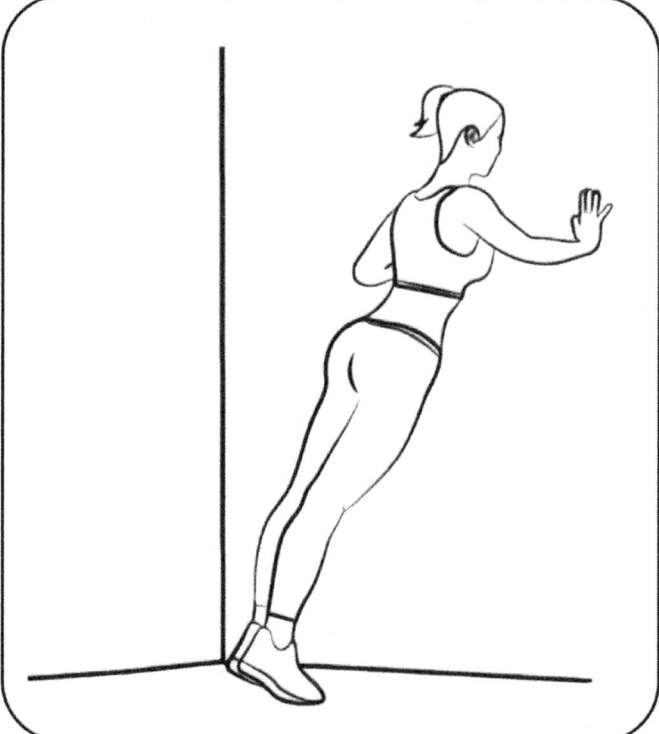

## Description

Wall Push-Ups are a variation of the classic floor push-ups. This exercise is ideal for strengthening the pectoral, deltoid, and triceps muscles, and it is also suitable for beginners or those with wrist problems.

**Execution:**
- Stand facing the wall, with your hands placed on the wall at shoulder level and your arms slightly bent.
- Tilt your torso toward the wall while bending your arms, bringing your chest closer to the wall.
- Push with your hands to return to the starting position.

**Breathing:**
- Inhaling, prepare for the descent.
- Exhaling, push with your hands toward the wall during the ascent phase.

**Benefits:**
- Strengthens chest, shoulder, and triceps muscles.
- Helps improve upper body stability.
- Safe and suitable variant even for those with wrist problems.

**Recommendations:**
- Keep your body in a straight line throughout the exercise, avoiding arching your back.
- Control the downward movement to avoid hitting the wall too quickly.
- If you have shoulder or wrist problems, consult a fitness professional or therapist before performing this exercise.

**Variants:**
- To make the exercise more intense, you can perform Wall Push-Ups with your hands lower than your shoulders.
- For an easier variation, you can move closer to the wall to reduce the amplitude of the downward movement.

# WALL ARM CIRCLES

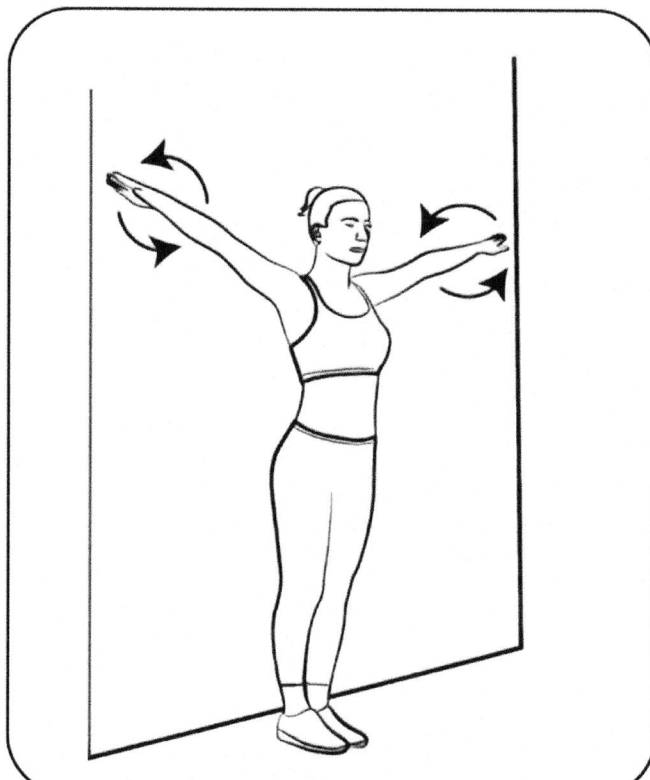 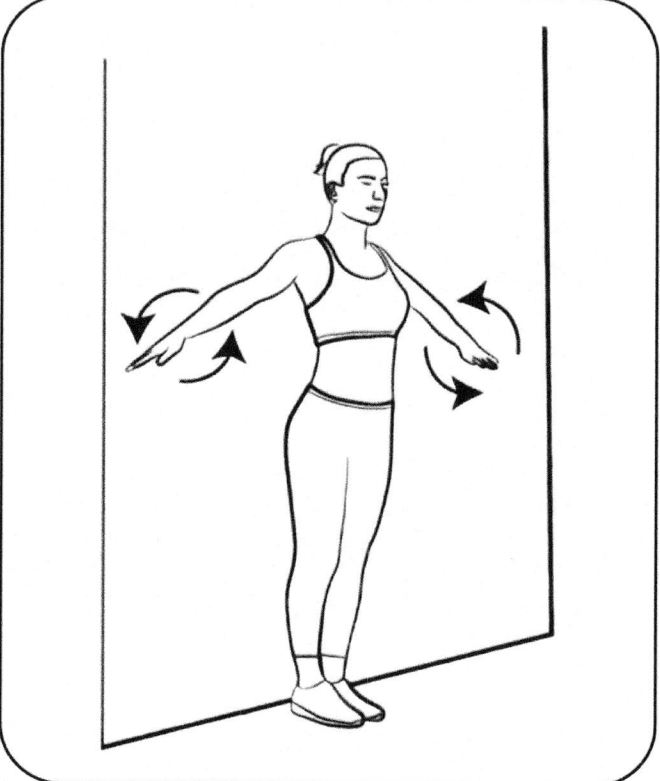

A Wall Arm Circle is a Pilates exercise that involves the upper limbs, helping to increase shoulder mobility and relax tension in the upper body. Using wall support, this exercise provides visual guidance for proper circular movement of the arms.

**Execution:**
- Stand facing the wall, with your arms extended sideways, parallel to the floor, and your hands resting on the wall surface at the same height as your shoulders.
- With your torso erect and shoulders relaxed, slowly begin to move your arms in outward circles, keeping your elbows slightly bent.
- Continue making circles with your arms clockwise for a few seconds, then change direction and make circles counterclockwise.
- Keep the movement fluid and controlled, focusing on shoulder mobility and lengthening arm muscles.

**Breathing:**
- Inhaling, prepare for circular, outward movement of arms.
- Exhaling, continue the circular motion, keeping the breath steady and regular.

**Benefits:**
- Increases the mobility of the shoulders and arms.
- Relaxes tension in the muscles of the arms and shoulders.
- Promotes better awareness of movement and posture.

**Recommendations:**
- Keep your torso erect and shoulders relaxed while performing the exercise.
- Avoid excessive pushing against the wall; keep the movement controlled and comfortable.

**Variants:**
- For a more intense variation, you can perform wider arm circles, thus increasing the intensity of the shoulder movement.
- For an easier variation, you can reduce the radius of the circles or perform the movement more slowly, thus reducing the intensity of arm and shoulder work.

# SINGLE ARM PUSH-UP

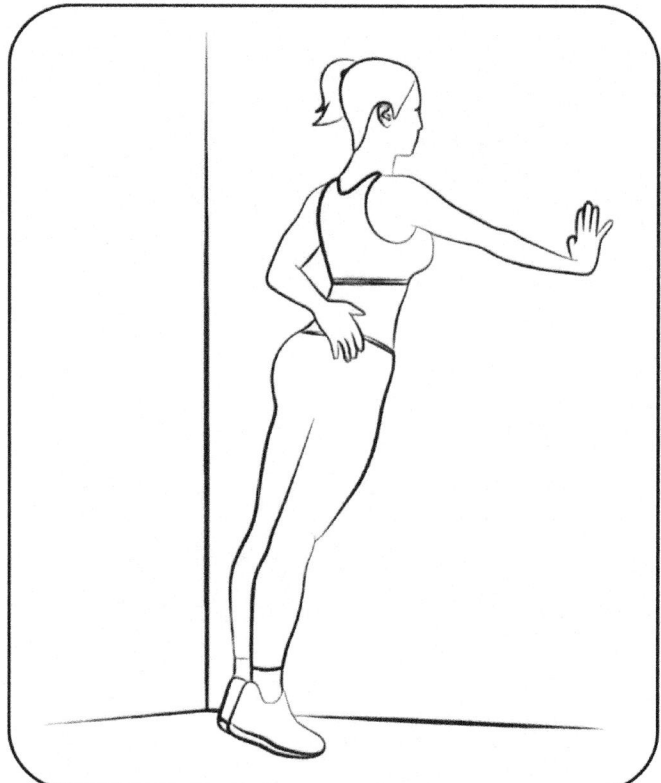 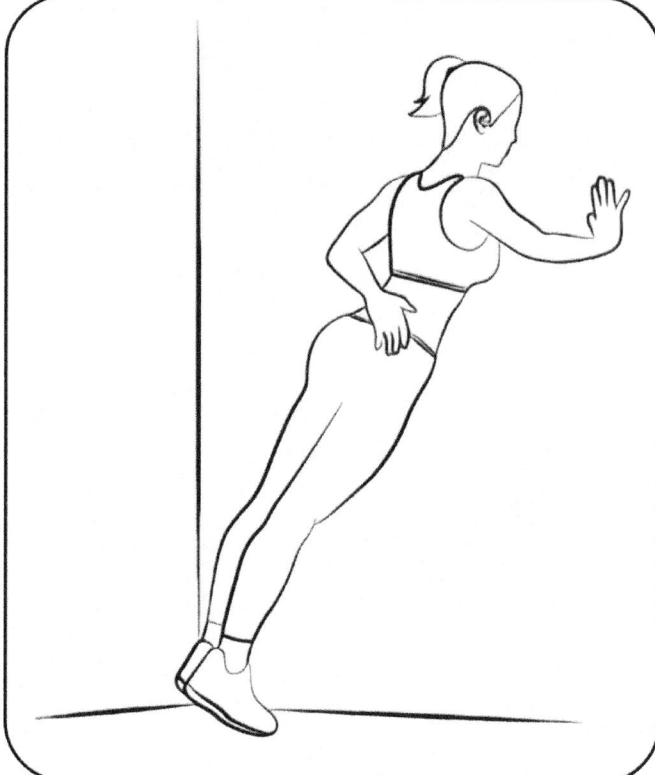

## Description

The Single Arm Push-Up is an advanced variation of the classic push-up that tests the strength and stability of the chest, shoulder and triceps muscles. This wall-based Pilates exercise requires a high level of core and arm strength to perform the movement with control and precision.

**Execution:**

- Stand in front of the wall with your hands resting on the wall at a slightly greater distance than your shoulders, aligned with your chest.
- Stretch your legs behind you, keeping your body aligned from head to toe, forming a straight line.
- Begin the movement by flexing one arm and slowly bending it toward the wall, lowering your chest until you touch the wall or get as close as possible.
- Keep the body in a stable and controlled position during the entire movement.
- Return to the starting position by extending your arm and pushing back until you reach the starting position.

**Breathing:**

- Inhaling, prepare for the exercise and hold a stable position.
- Exhaling, begin the arm flexion movement and lower the chest toward the wall.
- Continue to breathe rhythmically and in a controlled manner while performing.

**Benefits:**

- Requires high involvement of the core and arm muscles, thus helping to develop the strength and endurance of these muscle groups.
- Promotes improved stability and body control during pushing movements.
- Helps strengthen the chest, shoulders, triceps, and shoulder blade stabilizing muscles.

**Recommendations:**

- Before performing the Single Arm Push-Up, make sure you have a good foundation of strength and stability with traditional push-ups.
- Keep the body aligned throughout the movement and monitor the progress of arm flexion to avoid abrupt or incorrect movements.

**Variants:**

- To make the exercise easier, you can perform the Single Arm Push-Up with your knees resting on the floor instead of your legs extended.

## WALL SQUAT

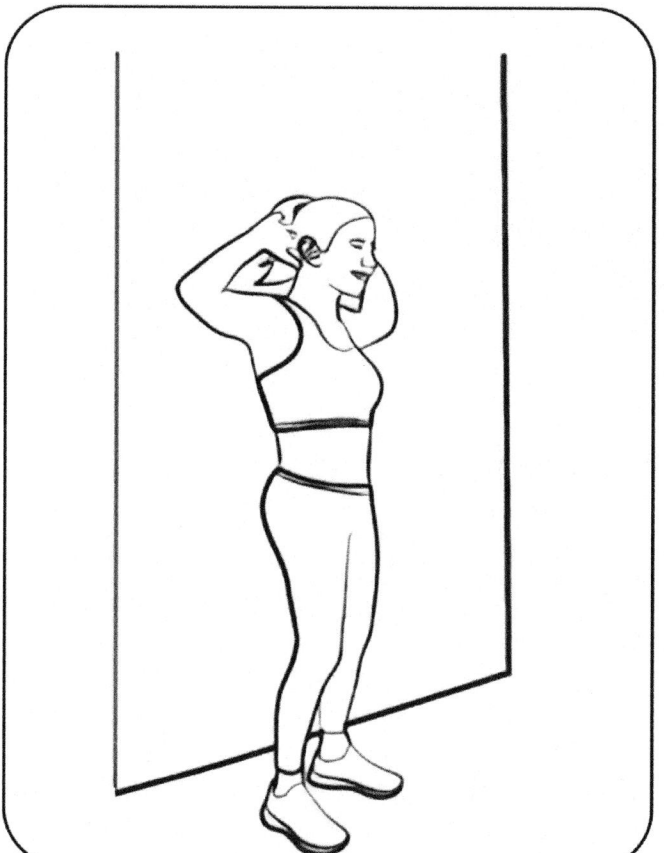 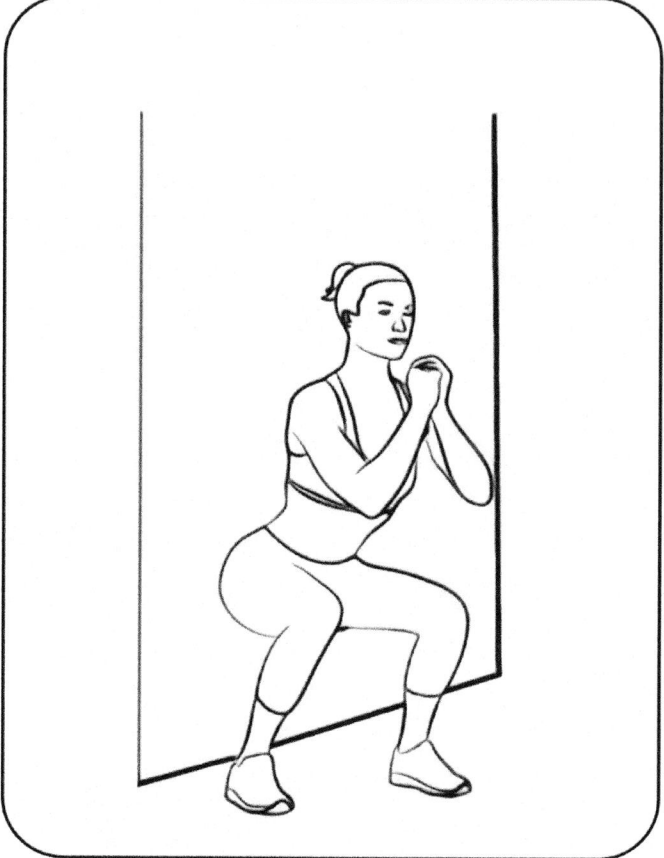

### Description

A Wall Squat is a Pilates exercise that aims to strengthen the lower limbs, particularly the quadriceps, glutes, and hip muscles. This position uses the support of the wall to provide stability during the exercise.

**Execution**:
- Position yourself with your back against the wall and your feet slightly apart, aligned with your shoulders.
- Drop into a squat position, bending your knees and lowering your hips downward.
- Keep your weight evenly distributed on both feet and make sure your knees are aligned with your ankles.
- Push your heels into the floor and return to a standing position.

**Breathing**:
- Inhaling, prepare for the downward movement.
- Exhaling, face the descent while maintaining smooth breathing during the entire movement.
- Inhaling again, rise back to a standing position.

**Benefits**:
- Strengthens leg and thigh muscles.
- Improves hip stability and joint mobility.
- Helps develop functional strength for daily activities.

**Recommendations**:
- Keep your back straight throughout the exercise, avoiding leaning forward.
- Be sure to keep your knees aligned with your ankles to avoid undue stress on your joints.
- If you have knee or hip problems, consult a fitness professional or therapist before performing this exercise.

**Variants**:
- For a more advanced variation, perform Wall Squats with your feet slightly further apart or trying to go even lower.
- For an easier variation, reduce the amplitude of the downward movement, keeping the movements controlled and precise.

## WALL SINGLE LEG SQUAT

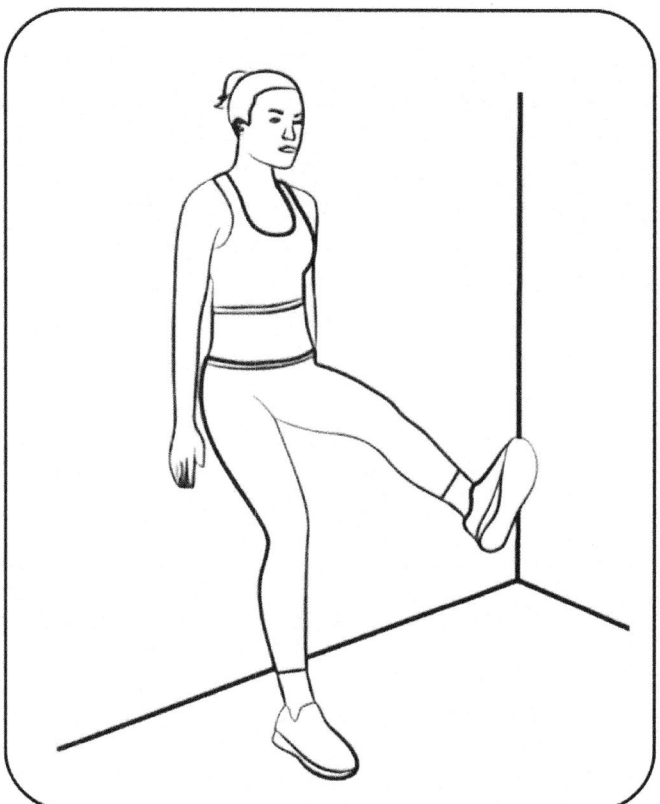 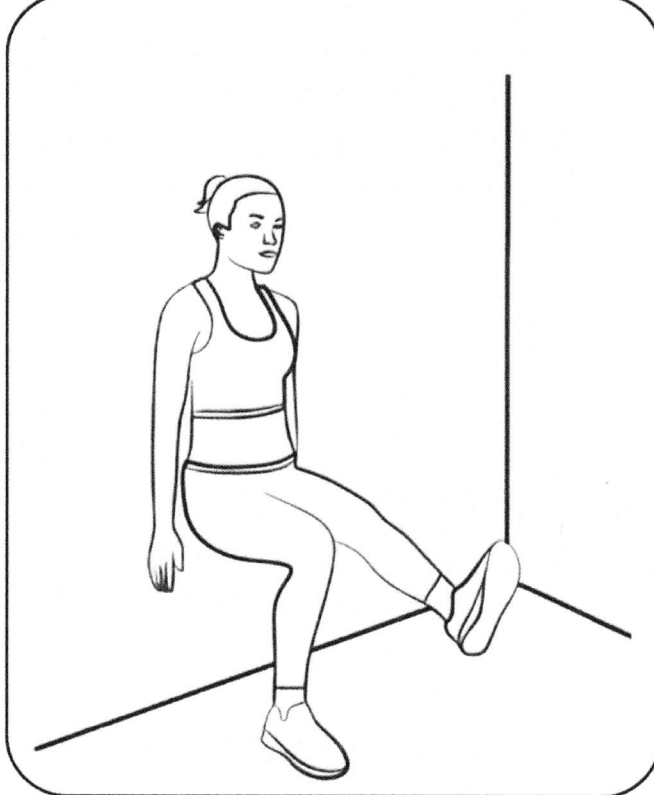

Wall Single Leg Squats are an advanced Pilates exercise that aims to improve lower limb strength and balance. Using wall support, this exercise allows you to focus on single limb work, developing the stability and strength needed to support the weight of the body on one leg.

**Execution**:
- Stand with your left side facing the wall.
- Place the palm of the left hand against the wall to maintain balance.
- Lift the right foot off the ground, bringing the knee up and bending it slightly.
- Inhaling, bend your left knee to lower into a lunge on your left leg, keeping your right foot lifted off the ground.
- Exhaling, push through the heel of the left leg to return to a standing position.
- Repeat the movement for a few repetitions, then switch sides and repeat on the other leg.

**Breathing**:
- Inhaling, prepare for the execution of the lunge on the left leg.
- Exhaling, push through the heel of the left leg to return to a standing position.

**Benefits**:
- Strengthens the leg muscles, particularly the quadriceps, ischiocrucials, and glutes.
- Improves balance and stability of the legs.
- Develops the functional strength needed to support the weight of the body on one leg.

**Recommendations**:
- Keep your torso upright while performing the lunge, avoiding leaning forward or backward.
- Focus on working the left leg muscles as you perform the lunge.
- If you have difficulty with balance, you can begin the exercise by using the support of a chair or cane.

**Variants**:
- For a more intense variation, you can hold your arms along your sides instead of resting your hand on the wall, increasing the challenge for balance.
- For an easier variation, you can perform Wall Single Leg Squats with the foot lifted only slightly off the ground, reducing the width of the lunge.

# WALL BRIDGE

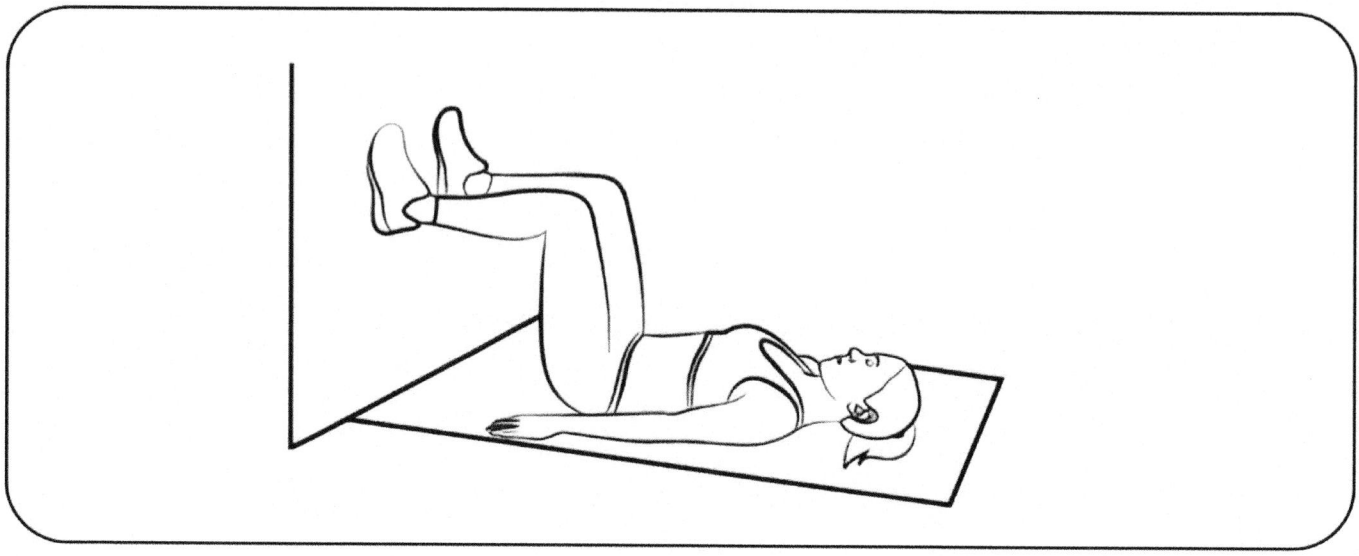

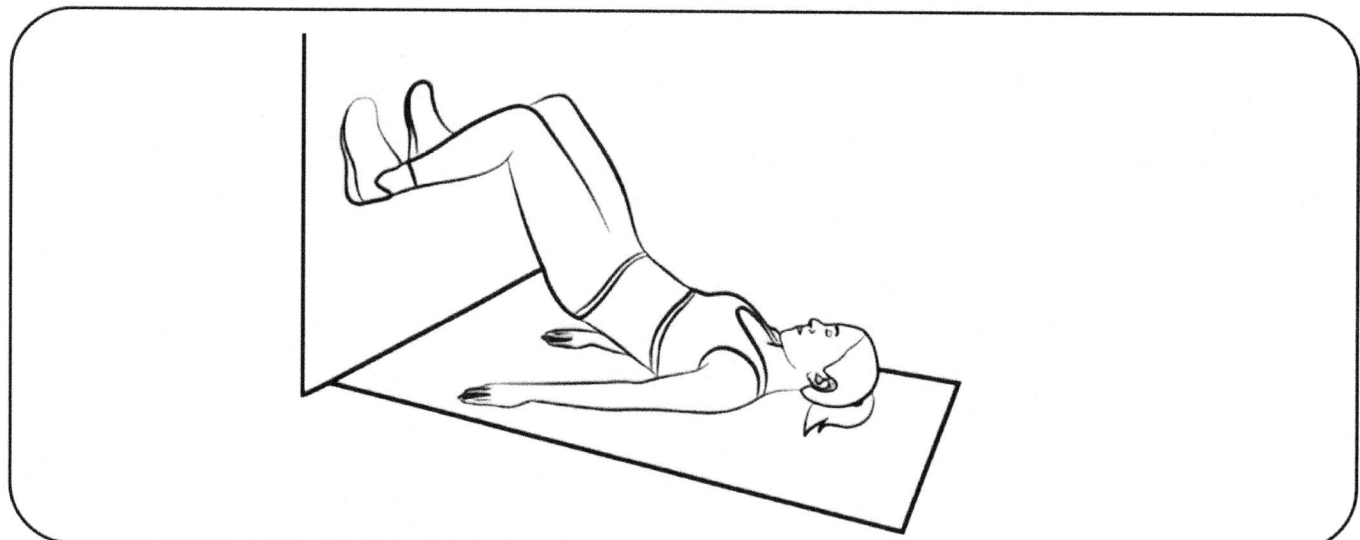

## Description

*The Wall Bridge is a Pilates exercise that works on strengthening the back, gluteal, and abdominal muscles. This position uses the support of the wall to provide stability while performing and allows you to work on realigning the spine.*

**Execution:**
- Lie on your back, with your legs bent and your feet resting against the wall.
- Arms should be relaxed at the sides of the body, palms facing downward.
- Push with your feet against the wall and lift your pelvis upward, forming a straight line from your shoulder to your knees.
- Hold the position for a few seconds, focusing on engaging the gluteal and abdominal muscles.
- Slowly release the pelvis toward the floor to return to the starting position.

**Breathing:**
- Inhaling, prepare for the pelvic lifting movement.
- As you exhale, lift your pelvis upward and maintain smooth breathing during the exercise.
- Inhaling again, slowly release the pelvis toward the floor.

**Benefits:**
- Strengthens the muscles of the legs, buttocks, and abdominals.
- Helps improve the alignment of the spine.
- Promotes stabilization of the pelvis and lower back.

**Recommendations:**
- Be sure to maintain a stable position during the exercise, avoiding rocking your pelvis.
- Do not overdo the flexion of the pelvis; avoid putting too much pressure on the lower back.
- If you have back or pelvic problems, consult a fitness professional or therapist before performing this exercise.

**Variants:**
- For a more intense variation, you can perform the Wall Bridge on one leg, keeping the other leg elevated in the air.
- For an easier variation, you can begin the exercise by lifting your pelvis only slightly off the floor. As you become more comfortable, you can increase the range of motion.

# WALL SINGLE LEG BRIDGE

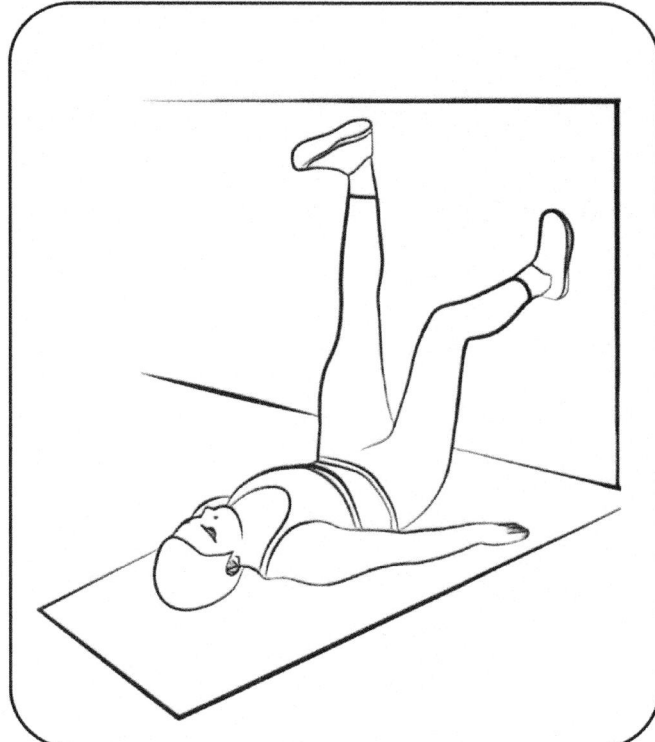 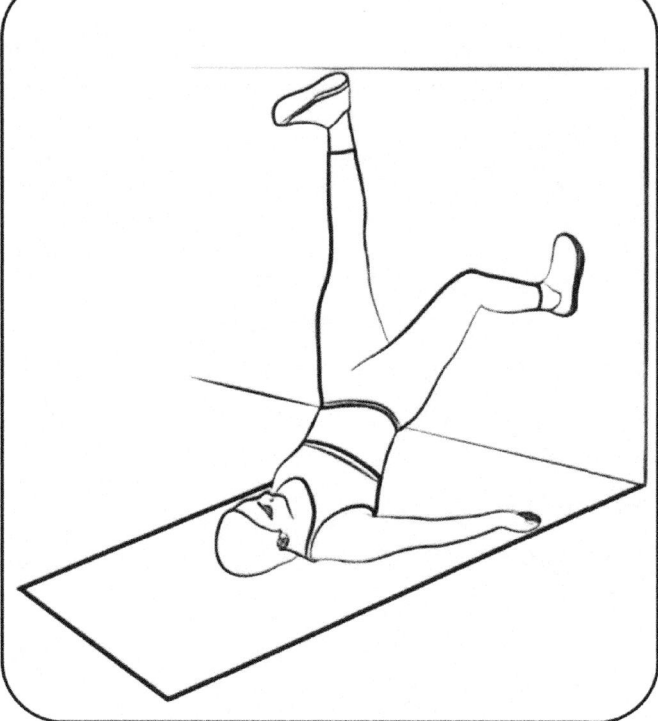

Wall Single Leg Bridge is a Pilates exercise that engages the core, glutes and upper body muscles. It uses the wall support to provide stability while performing, allowing you to focus on alignment and specific involvement of the muscles involved.

**Execution**:
- Position yourself on the floor with your legs toward the wall.
- Place one foot against the wall, maintaining adequate distance to allow the pelvis to lift.
- Extend your arms along your sides, with your palms facing downward and your fingers pointing toward your feet.
- Inhaling, lift the pelvis off the floor and extend the other leg upward, forming a straight line between the shoulders and knees.
- Hold the raised position for a few seconds, trying to activate the glutes and core muscles.
- Exhaling, slowly lower the pelvis back to the starting position.

**Breathing**:
- Inhaling, prepare for the pelvic lifting movement.
- Exhaling, lift the pelvis off the floor.
- Inhaling again, hold the raised position for a few seconds.
- Exhaling, slowly lower the pelvis back to the starting position.

**Benefits**:
- Strengthens core muscles, particularly the glutes, abdominals, and lower back.
- Promotes proper alignment of the spine and improves the stability of the spine.
- Improves flexibility of the spine and hips.

**Recommendations**:
- Keep your neck and shoulders relaxed while performing the exercise.
- Focus on contracting your glutes and core muscles as you lift your pelvis.

**Variants**:
- For an easier variation, you can perform the Wall Bridge with both feet resting on the wall.

# WALL LEG CIRCLE

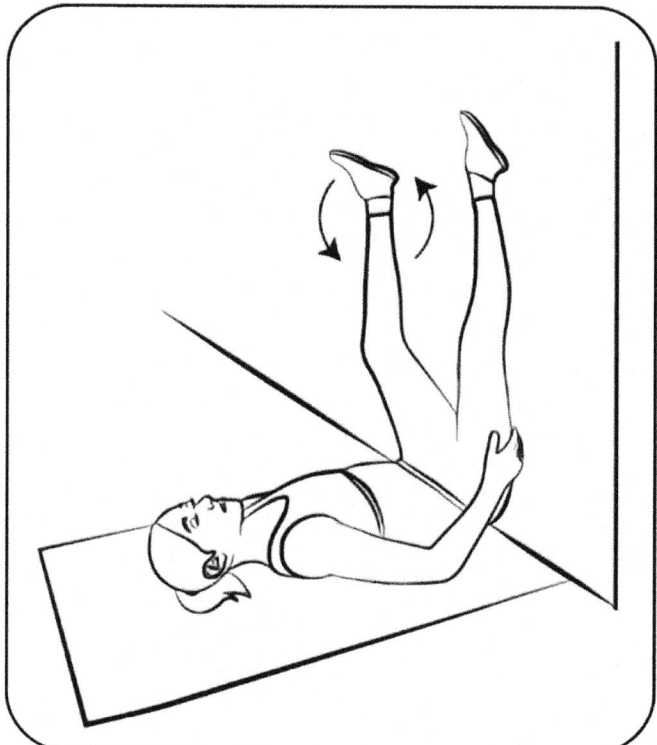 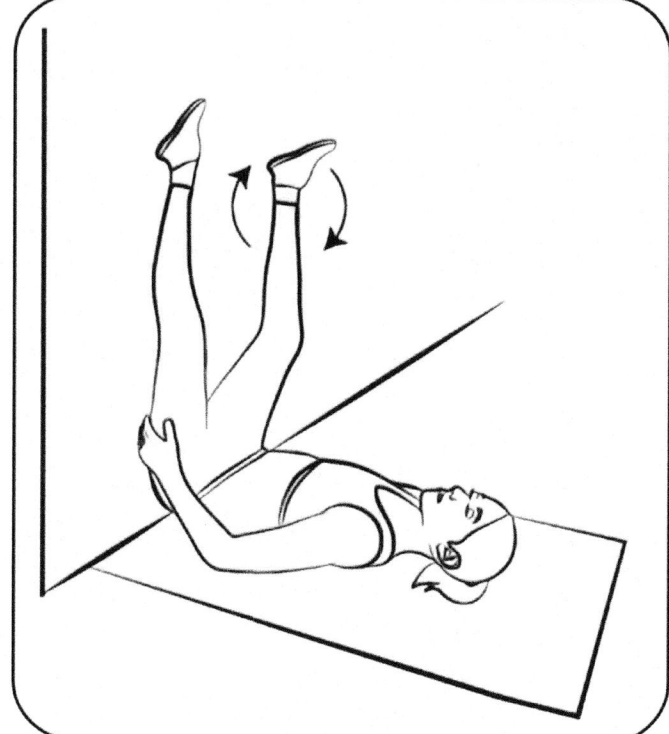

A Wall Leg Circle is a Pilates exercise that aims to strengthen and increase the flexibility of the legs and abs. Using the wall support, this exercise allows you to perform controlled circles with your legs, engaging different muscle groups.

**Execution:**
- Position yourself lying on the floor, with your buttocks and lower back against the wall.
- Lift both legs off the floor and stretch them vertically against the wall.
- Start by running circles with your legs, keeping your lower back and glutes in contact with the wall.
- You can perform the circles either clockwise or counterclockwise.
- Make a few circles in one direction and then change directions to complete the set.

**Breathing:**
- Breathing in, prepare for the movement of circles with the legs.
- Exhaling, control the movement as you draw circles with your legs.

**Benefits:**
- Strengthens abdominal and leg muscles.
- Increases hip and leg flexibility.
- Improves coordination and body stability.

**Recommendations:**
- Keep your lower back pressed against the wall while performing the exercise.
- Perform controlled circles with the legs without moving the pelvis or shoulders.

**Variants:**
- For a more intense variation, you can use weighted ankle straps or elastic bands to increase the resistance of the movement.
- For an easier variation, you can perform smaller circles with your legs or keep one of your legs resting on the floor while doing circles with the other leg.

# WALL LUNGES

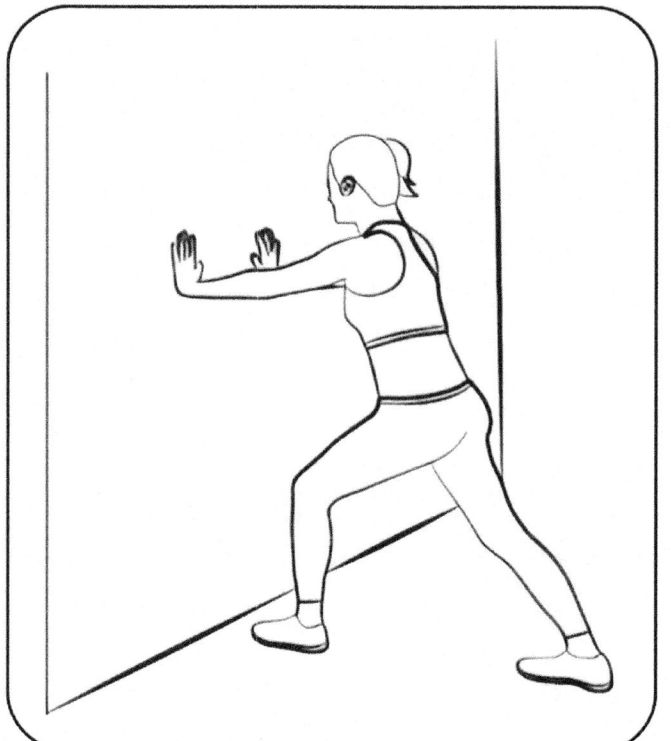 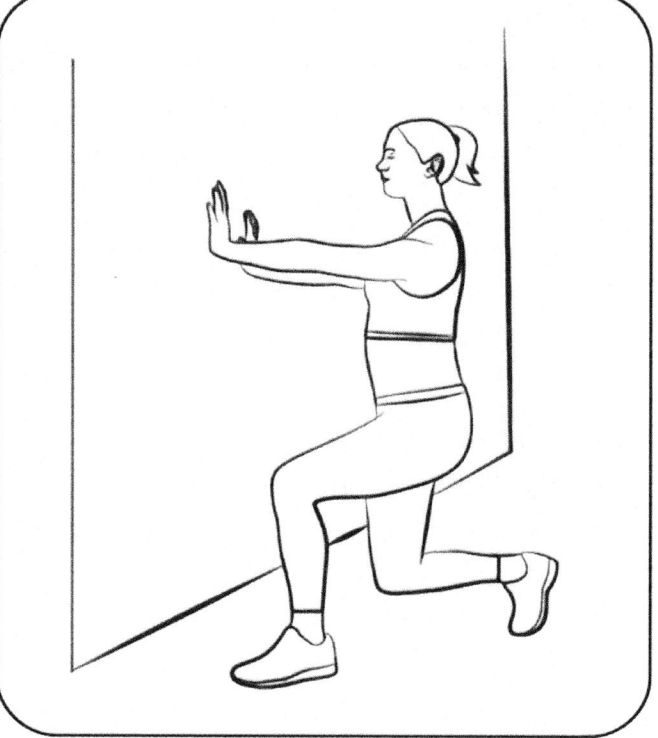

A Wall Lunge is a Pilates exercise that involves the lower limbs, particularly the leg and gluteal muscles. Using the support of the wall, this exercise provides stability and aid in the proper execution of the lunge position.

**Execution**:
- Stand facing the wall, with your hands resting on the wall surface at the same height as your shoulders.
- Step backward with your right foot, moving away from the wall, while your left foot stays forward.
- Bend both knees, lowering your pelvis toward the floor and forming two 90-degree angles with your legs (one leg backward and the other forward).
- Make sure the front knee is aligned above the ankle and the back knee to ankle is parallel to the floor.
- Keep your torso erect and your shoulders relaxed, avoiding leaning forward.
- Hold the position for a few seconds, then return to the starting position and repeat the exercise with the other leg.

**Breathing**:
- Inhaling, prepare for the lunge movement.
- Exhaling, bend the knees and lower the pelvis into the lunge position.
- Inhaling, hold the lunge position.
- Exhaling, return to the starting position.

**Benefits**:
- Strengthens the muscles of the legs, buttocks, and core.
- Improves balance and stability.
- Promotes improved flexibility of the legs and hips.

**Recommendations**:
- Be sure to keep your back straight and shoulders relaxed while performing the exercise.
- Don't push too hard against the wall; keep the movement controlled and comfortable.

**Variants**:
- For a more intense variation, you can add weights to your hands to increase resistance during the lunge.
- For an easier variation, you can reduce the depth of the lunge by bending your knees slightly.

# WALL SCISSORS

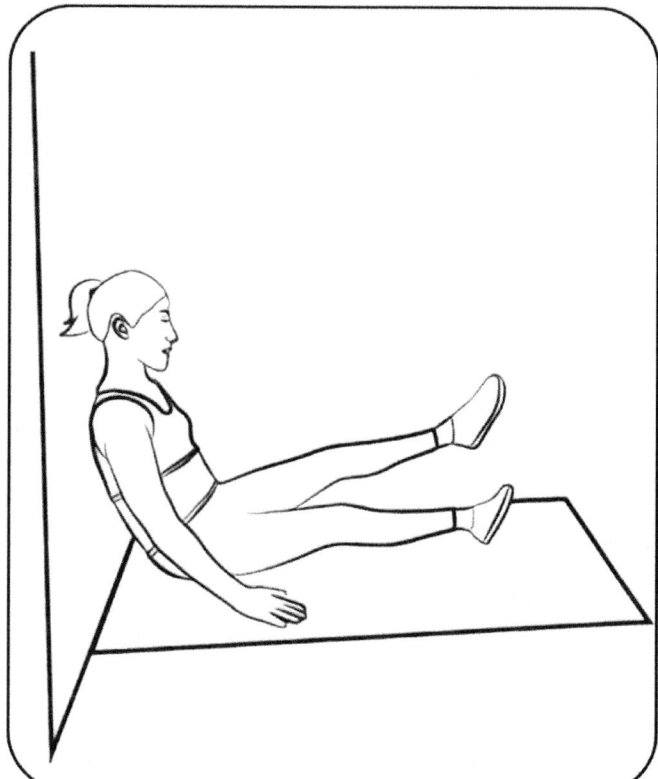 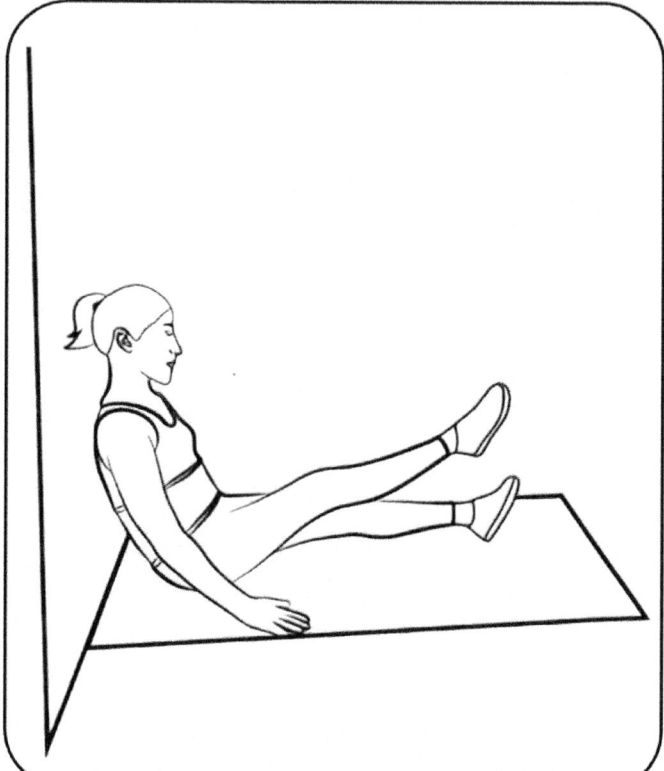

Description

A Wall Scissor is a Pilates exercise that involves the lower limbs and core. Using wall support, this exercise provides stability and aid in the proper execution of leg movement.

**Execution:**
- Sit with your back resting against the wall, legs extended, and your hands resting on the floor.
- Lift both legs off the floor, keeping them taut and parallel to the floor.
- Begin performing a scissor motion with your legs, bringing one leg up and one leg down without touching the floor.
- Continue to perform the movement alternately, sliding the legs back and forth like scissors.

**Breathing:**
- Inhaling, prepare for the leg scissor movement.
- Exhaling, begin the scissor movement, keeping the breath steady and regular during execution.

**Benefits:**
- Strengthens leg muscles, particularly the quadriceps.
- Improves coordination and balance.
- Activates the core, involving the abdominals and lower back muscles.

**Recommendations:**
- Keep your torso erect and shoulders relaxed while performing the exercise.
- Focus on controlling leg movement and core stability.

**Variants:**
- For a more intense variation, you can add a heavy anklet to your legs to increase resistance during the scissor movement.
- For an easier variation, you can perform the scissors movement with your legs slightly bent or rest only one leg at a time on the floor for more support.

# WALL SIDE LEG LIFTS

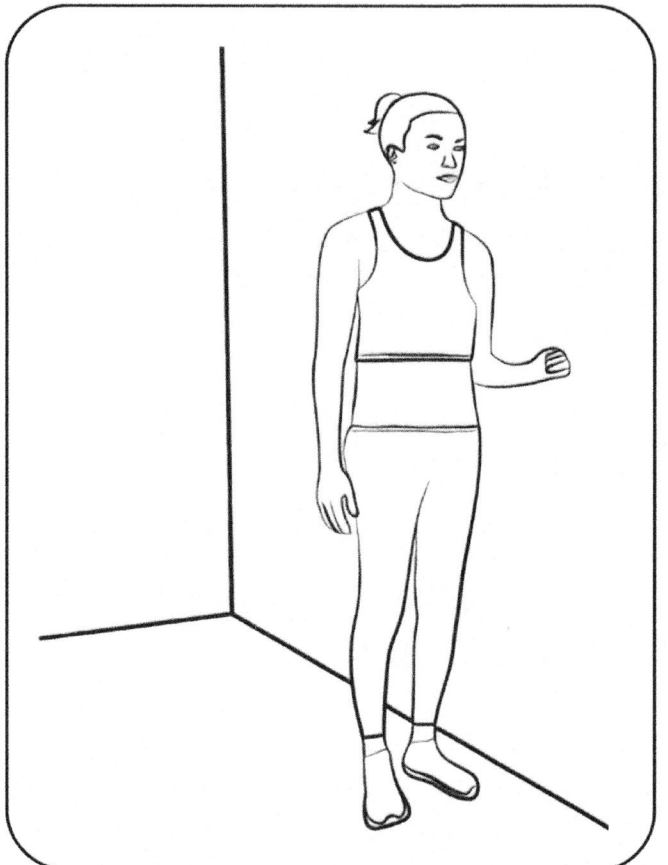 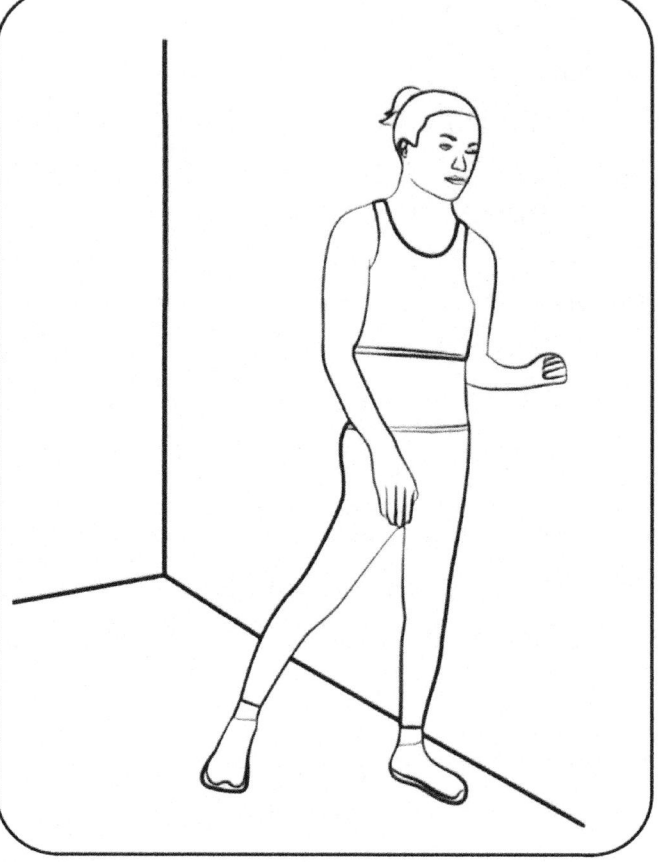

### Description

A Wall Side Leg Lift is a Pilates exercise focused on strengthening and toning the side muscles of the legs and hip. Using the wall for support, this exercise provides stability and allows for controlled movement.

**Execution**:
- Stand sideways to the wall, with your hip and forearm resting against the wall.
- Make sure the body is aligned from head to toe, with the elbow under the shoulder and the hip resting fully against the wall.
- Align the feet and legs, maintaining slight knee flexion for stability.
- Inhaling, prepare for the lateral leg lift.
- Exhaling, slowly lift the leg upward.
- Maintain the leg-lift position.
- Slowly return the leg to the starting position.

**Breathing**:
- Inhaling, prepare for the lateral leg lift.
- Exhaling, lift the leg in a controlled manner.
- Inhaling, hold the lifting position, breathing deeply to maintain control.
- Exhaling, slowly bring the leg back to the starting position.

**Benefits**:
- Strengthens and tones the lateral muscles of the legs and hip.
- Promotes balance and stability of the body.
- Improves body awareness and coordination.

**Recommendations**:
- Keep the body stable and aligned while performing the exercise, avoiding protruding the pelvis or bending the back.
- Maintain a light abdominal contraction to stabilize the core during the movement.

**Variants**:
- For a more intense variation, you can perform the exercise by holding a heavy anklet on your raised leg.
- For an easier variation, you can perform the exercise by reducing the range of motion and keeping the leg slightly bent.

## MOUNTAIN CLIMBER WALL

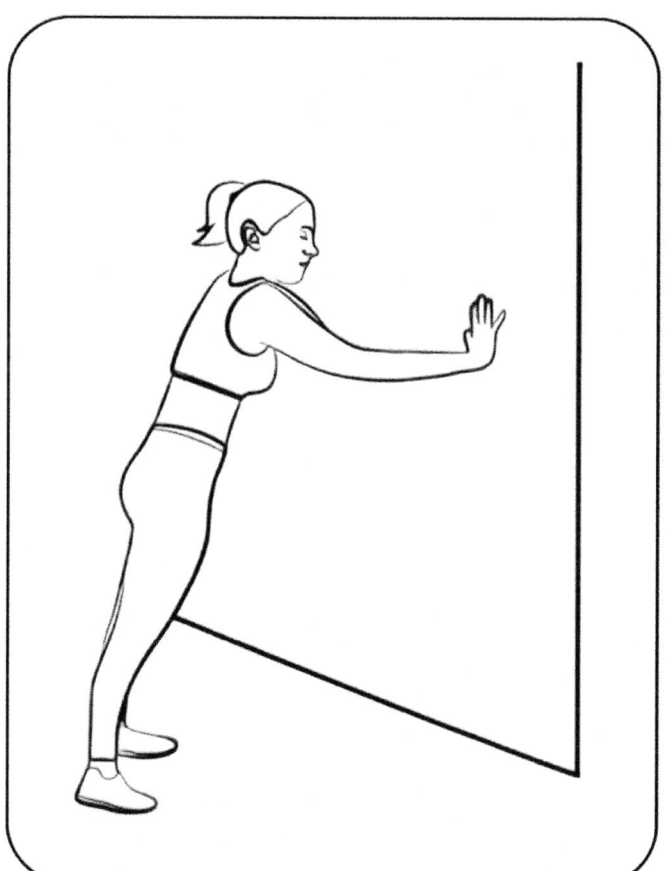 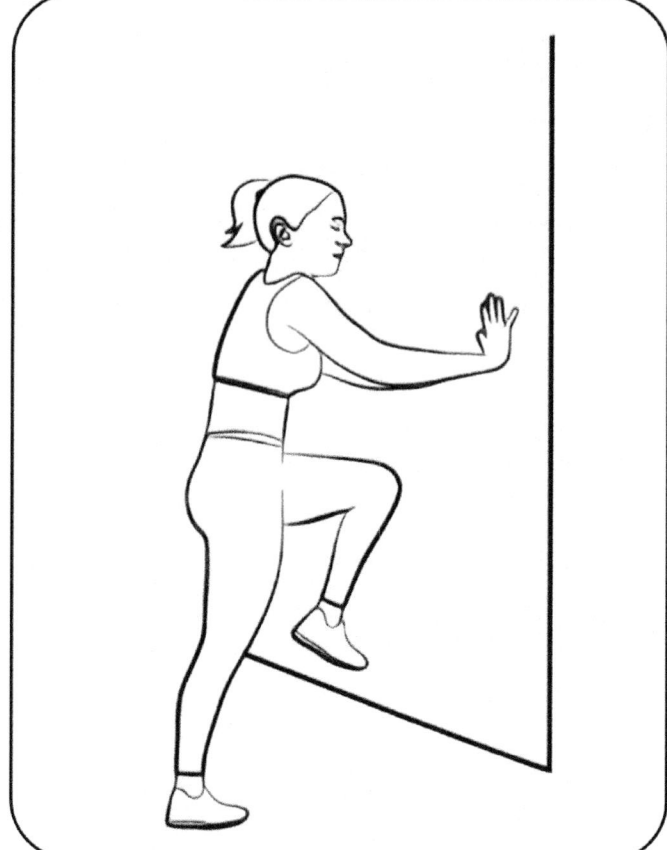

### Description

The Mountain Climber Wall is a dynamic Pilates wall exercise that involves the abdominals, arms, and legs. This variation of the classic mountain climber is performed with the hands resting on the wall and involves running in place to increase the intensity of the workout.

**Execution**:
- Stand facing the wall with your arms outstretched and your hands resting on the wall, aligned with your shoulders.
- Move your torso slightly away from the wall while keeping your arms extended and your body in a prone plank position.
- Step backward with one foot, keeping the body aligned from neck to heels.
- Once in the mountain climber position, start performing a run in place by alternately bringing your knees as close to your chest as possible, as if you were climbing a mountain.
- Continue to perform the movement alternately and dynamically for the duration of the exercise.

**Breathing**:
- Inhaling, prepare for the movement by maintaining a relaxed posture.
- Exhaling, start performing the run in place by alternately bringing the knees toward the chest.
- Keep breathing rhythmically during the exercise.

**Benefits**:
- Involves many muscle groups, including the abdominals, arms, legs, and stabilizing muscles of the trunk.
- Helps improve strength and endurance of the lower and upper limbs.
- Promotes coordination and core stabilization ability.

**Recommendations**:
- Maintain correct posture while performing, avoiding lifting the hips or sinking the shoulders.
- Keep your abs tightly contracted to support your trunk and protect your back.
- Perform the exercise dynamically, keeping a steady pace while running in place.

**Variants**:
- If you need an easier variation, you can perform the Mountain Climber Wall by keeping your hands resting on a higher surface, such as a bench or chair, instead of the wall.
- To increase the intensity, you can try performing the mountain climber faster or adding an alternating jump between the legs during the movement.

# WALL SIT

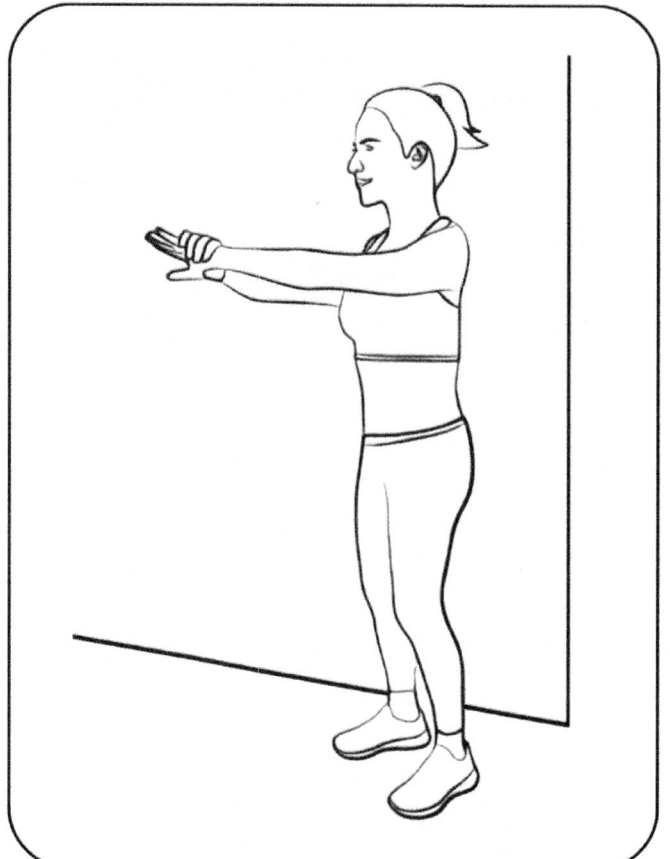 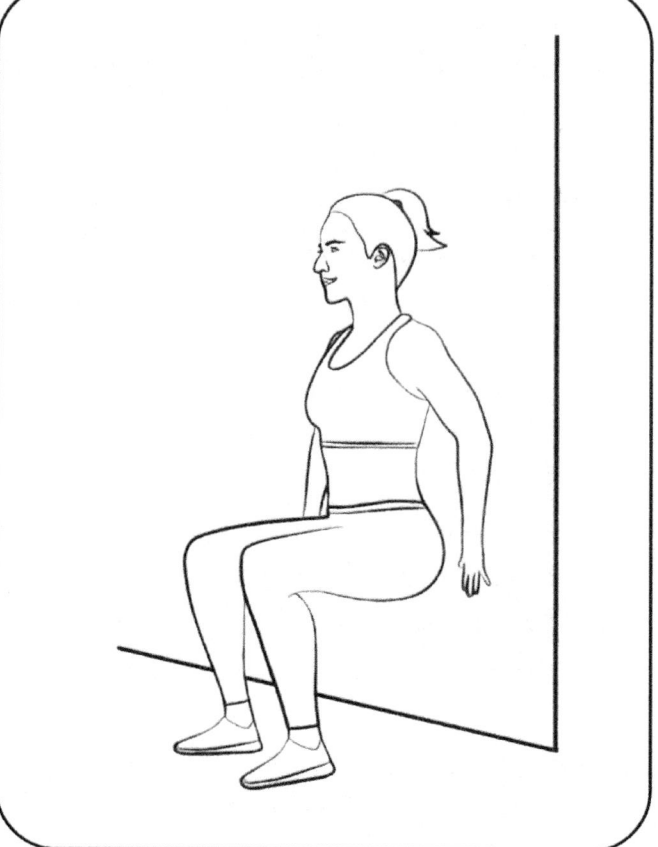

The Wall Sit is a wall Pilates exercise that primarily involves the leg, gluteal, and core muscles. This static position is ideal for improving muscle strength and endurance in the lower extremities.

**Execution:**
- Stand facing away from the wall with your feet a little further apart than your shoulders.
- Step forward and lean back slightly against the wall, keeping your back straight and in contact with the vertical surface.
- Begin descending in a squat motion, bending the knees until they form an angle of about 90 degrees. Your knees should be aligned with your ankles and thighs parallel to the floor.
- Keep your body weight on your heels and arms stretched forward to maintain balance.
- Hold this position for the desired length of time or the recommended number of repetitions.

**Breathing:**
- Inhaling, prepare for the exercise and hold a relaxed position.
- Exhaling, begin to descend in a squat motion against the wall.
- Continue to breathe rhythmically and in a controlled manner while performing.

Benefits:
- Develops lower limb strength, including the thigh, gluteal, and calf muscles.
- Promotes improved balance and core stability.
- Helps tone leg muscles and helps improve muscular endurance.

**Recommendations:**
- Keep your back firmly against the wall throughout the execution to support the spine and reduce stress on the joints.
- Be sure to keep your knees aligned with your ankles and your body weight on your heels to avoid overloading your knees.
- Avoid bending your back or leaning your torso forward; maintain a straight and aligned posture.

**Variants:**
- To make the exercise easier, you can reduce the time you stay in the position or perform shallower squats.
- To increase the intensity, you can hold the position for a longer period or use weights to increase resistance.

# BACK LEG LIFT

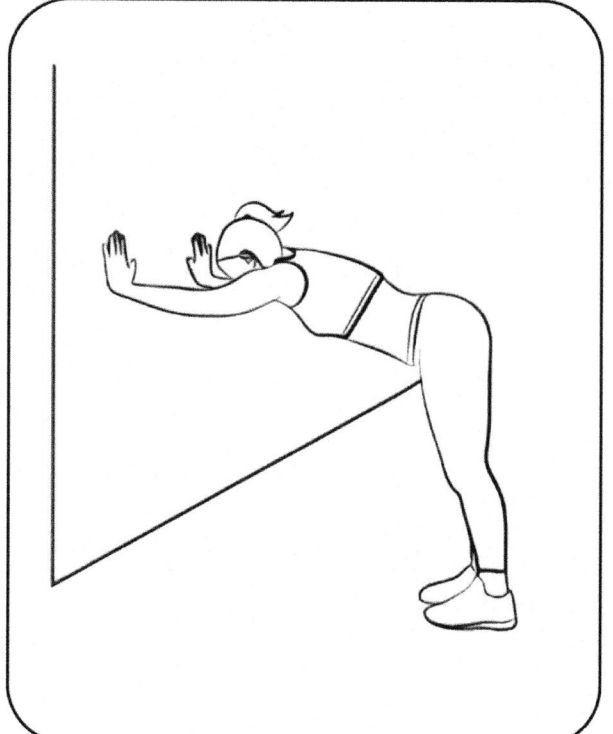 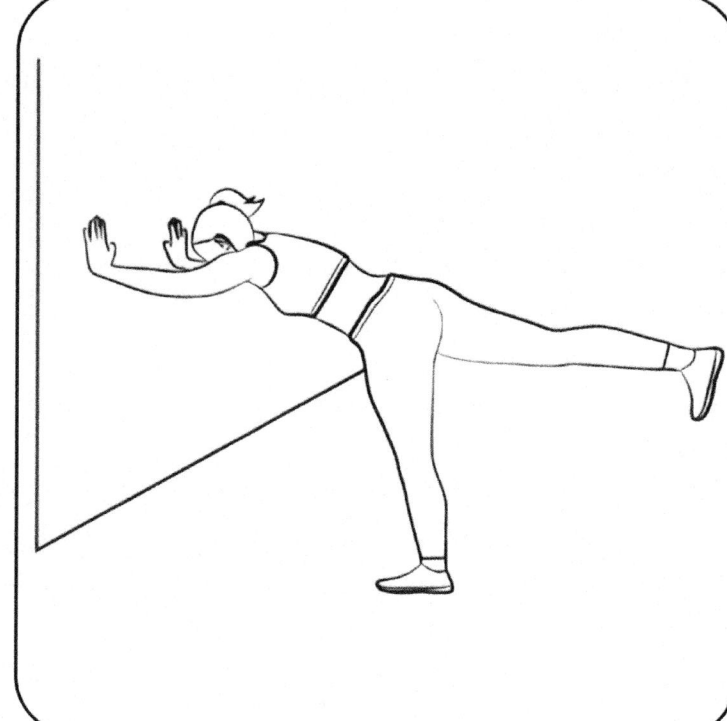

The Back Leg Lift is a wall Pilates exercise aimed at strengthening the muscles of the back of the body, particularly the glutes and back muscles. This movement helps improve stability, balance, and coordination, helping to create a more upright posture and greater functional strength.

68

**Execution**:

- Stand facing the wall with your feet aligned at shoulder height. Tilt your torso forward, forming an angle of about 90 degrees with your legs.
- Rest your hands on the wall at about shoulder height and stretch your arms forward.
- Begin the execution by lifting one of the legs backward, forming a straight line parallel to the floor between the hands and the lifted foot.
- Keep your torso and hip stable during the movement and contract your glutes to lift your leg in a controlled manner.
- Return to the starting position by lowering the leg and repeat the exercise with the other leg.

**Breathing**:

- Inhaling, prepare for the exercise by maintaining a stable and controlled posture.
- Exhaling, lift the leg backward by contracting the glutes and keeping the torso tilted forward.
- Keep breathing smoothly and with control throughout the exercise.

**Benefits**:

- Strengthens the muscles of the back of the body, particularly the glutes, back muscles, and stabilizing muscles of the spine.
- Helps improve balance and coordination because it requires high involvement of the stabilizing muscles during execution.
- Promotes improved posture and body alignment, helping to prevent postural problems and lower back pain.

**Recommendations**:

- While performing, keep your torso tilted forward and your core contracted to ensure proper activation of the muscles in the back of the body.
- Control the leg movement throughout the execution and avoid lifting the leg too high to avoid undue tension on the back.

**Variants**:

- To make the exercise easier, you can perform the Back Leg Lift with your hands resting on a higher surface, such as a bench or chair, thus reducing the angle at which your torso is tilted.
- To increase the intensity, you can use elastic bands tied to your ankles to create more resistance while performing the movement.

# HEALTHY EATING

Nutrition plays a key role in achieving your weight loss goals and overall health improvement. By combining proper nutrition with Pilates wall training, you can maximize results and achieve sustainable weight loss over time. This sub-chapter will provide a guide to balanced nutrition and conscious food choices to promote weight loss in combination with Pilates on the wall.

1. **Balanced nutrition**:
   A balanced diet is essential to provide the body with the nutrients it needs to function properly and to support wall Pilates training. Here are some key principles of balanced nutrition:

   - Consume a variety of foods: Be sure to include a wide range of nutritious foods in your diet, such as fruits, vegetables, whole grains, lean proteins, and sources of healthy fats. This will provide you with a full range of essential nutrients.

   - Balance macronutrients: Try to balance the intake of carbohydrates, protein, and fat in your diet. Carbohydrates, found in whole grains such as quinoa, spelt, and oats, provide sustained energy. Lean proteins, such as those found in chicken, fish, and legumes, aid in muscle repair and recovery. Healthy fats, such as those found in avocados, nuts, and olive oil, are important for overall health.

   - Limit sugars and highly processed foods: Minimize consumption of added sugars and highly processed foods, such as sugary drinks, sweets, packaged snacks, and fried foods. These foods are often high in empty calories and low in essential nutrients.

2. **Conscious food choices**:
   In addition to following a balanced diet, it is important to make conscious food choices that support your weight loss goal. Here are some helpful suggestions:
   - Control portions: Pay attention to portion sizes and try to eat mindfully. Learn to recognize your feelings of fullness and stop when you are satisfied.

   - Eat slowly: Take the time to eat slowly and savor each bite. This will help you feel fuller and avoid overeating.

- Drink enough: Maintain adequate hydration by drinking enough water throughout the day. Water helps regulate appetite and maintain energy during exercise.

- Choose whole, fresh foods: Focus on choosing whole, unprocessed foods. Opt for whole grains such as quinoa, spelt, and oats instead of refined products. Choose lean meats, such as chicken, turkey, or fish, instead of processed meats. Prefer sources of healthy fats, such as avocados, olive oil, and nuts, rather than foods high in saturated fats.

- Pay attention to snacks: Choose healthy and nutritious snacks, such as fresh fruit, nuts, seeds, or low-fat yogurt. Avoid snacks that are high in calories and low in nutrients.

- Balance the colors on your plate: Try to create colorful, nutrient-rich dishes. Choose a variety of fruits and vegetables of different colors to get a full range of antioxidants, vitamins, and minerals. Include dark green leafy vegetables, such as spinach and kale, and various types of seafood, such as salmon or tuna, to benefit from omega-3 fatty acids.

- Use herbs and spices: To add flavor to your dishes, experiment with a variety of herbs and spices. In addition to making meals tastier, many herbs and spices also have health benefits. For example, turmeric, ginger, garlic, and cayenne pepper may have anti-inflammatory and antioxidant properties.

- ncorporate fiber-rich foods: Dietary fiber is important for digestive health, bowel regularity, and feeling full. Include fiber-rich foods such as legumes, whole grains, fruits, vegetables, and seeds in your diet. These foods can help control appetite and keep blood sugar levels stable.

3. **Balance and flexibility**:
Remember that a balanced diet does not mean deprivation or excessive restriction. It is important to find a balance that allows you to enjoy even your favorite foods in moderation. Flexibility in dieting is essential to maintain a healthy relationship with food and to ensure long-term, sustainable weight loss.

4. **Meal preparation**:
Take time to prepare meals in advance to simplify your eating during the week. Prepare large portions of foods such as grilled chicken, steamed vegetables, or

whole grains and store them in sealed containers in the refrigerator to have them ready when you need them. This way, you will avoid relying on convenience foods or less healthy temptations when you are in a hurry.

5. **Listen to your body**:

Develop a greater awareness of your body and its needs. Learn to distinguish between physical hunger and emotional hunger, to satisfy your appetite with nutritious foods, and to stop when you are satisfied. Pay attention to your body's hunger and satiety signals and adjust your diet accordingly.

Here are some practical suggestions for dealing with this problem:

- Identify your emotions: Before you give in to emotional hunger, it is important to take a moment to identify the emotions you are experiencing. Emotional hunger often manifests as a response to a negative emotional state, such as stress, sadness, or boredom. Being aware of your emotions helps you recognize when the hunger you are experiencing is not due to a real need for nourishment, but rather is a response to an emotional state. Identifying your emotions is the first step in dealing with them more consciously.

- Practice food awareness: Food awareness is a practice that helps you connect with your body, pay attention to physical sensations, and recognize hunger and satiety signals. When it comes to dealing with emotional hunger, food awareness becomes even more important. Learn to eat slowly, savoring each bite and observing how food makes you feel. Ask yourself if you are eating to satisfy a real need for nourishment or if you are trying to compensate for a negative emotion. Food awareness helps you distinguish between physical hunger and emotional hunger, enabling you to make more informed choices about food.

- Keep a food and emotional diary: Keeping a food and emotional diary can be a great strategy for better understanding your eating habits and connections to emotions. Record what you eat, when you eat it, and how you feel at the time. This helps you identify any patterns or associations between your emotions and eating. For example, you might notice that when you feel stressed, you have a tendency to eat foods high in sugar. Identifying these connections helps you become aware of your eating behaviors and find alternative strategies for managing emotions without resorting to food.

- Develop a list of healthy alternatives: When you feel the temptation to give in to emotional hunger, it is helpful to have a list of healthy alternatives available that you can adopt instead of food. These alternatives can be activities you enjoy that help you distract yourself or manage your emotions in a healthier way. For example, you could try taking a walk outdoors, engaging in a creative hobby, listening to relaxing music, practicing meditation, or reading an interesting book. Find what works best for you and create a list of activities that allow you to satisfy the need for gratification or distraction without resorting to food.

- Practice stress management techniques: Stress is often a major cause of emotional hunger. Learning stress management techniques will help you reduce the likelihood of turning to food as a compensatory mechanism. There are several techniques you can try, such as deep breathing, yoga, meditation, or progressive muscle relaxation training. Experiment with these techniques and find the one that helps you reduce stress and manage your emotions in a more balanced way.

- Seek social support: Coping with emotional hunger can be a challenge, but you are not alone. Seek support from friends, family, or an online community that shares your wellness goals. Sharing your experiences, successes, and struggles with others can offer a sense of support and encouragement. You might also consider the help of a wellness professional, such as a nutritionist or emotional eating counselor, who can provide you with personalized strategies to address emotional hunger and achieve your health and wellness goals.

Nutrition is an essential component in achieving your weight loss goals in conjunction with wall Pilates training. Experiment, listen to your body, and work with a nutrition professional to create a personalized nutrition plan that fits your specific needs and goals.

# CHALLENGES AND SOLUTIONS

## Motivation and Plateaus

During a weight loss program, it is natural to encounter challenges along the way. No matter how strong your resolve, there will be times when you may feel unmotivated or experience a lack of progress. This sub-chapter will provide tips for dealing with some of the most common challenges you may encounter during your weight loss journey, particularly lack of motivation and plateaus.

Lack of motivation is a common experience for many people trying to lose weight. You may start out with great enthusiasm, but over time, you may feel discouraged or unmotivated. It is important to understand that lack of motivation is normal and can affect anyone. Do not let this lack of motivation stop you in your weight loss journey. There are several strategies you can adopt to deal with this challenge and regain motivation:

- Set realistic and specific goals:
  Set weight loss goals that are realistic and specific to you. Setting short-term goals that are achievable will help you maintain motivation and a sense of progress. For example, instead of focusing only on the total weight you want to lose, focus your attention on smaller goals, such as improving your physical endurance, increasing the number of repetitions of a particular exercise, or achieving a certain number of weekly workouts.

- Find your "why:"
  Identify the deep reasons why you want to lose weight and improve your health. Ask yourself what your personal "why" is. This could be related to your health, self-esteem, increased energy, or a desire to improve your quality of life. Keeping your "why" in mind will help you maintain motivation during difficult times and overcome obstacles along the way.

- Create a supportive environment:
  Seek the support of friends and family who will encourage and support you during your weight loss program. Try to avoid negative influences and try to surround yourself with people who inspire you and help you stay motivated. If necessary, also seek out support groups or professionals in the field, such as nutritionists or fitness consultants, who can offer you additional support and guidance.

- Find a training partner or support group:
  Sharing the journey with someone can be extremely motivating. Find a friend or training partner with whom you can share goals, challenges, and victories. Set up training sessions together, exchange advice and encouragement, and hold each other accountable. If you can't find a workout partner, join online groups or participate in communities of fitness enthusiasts where you can share your experiences and get support.

- Visualize your goals:
  Creating a clear and vivid vision of your goals can help you maintain motivation. Use tools such as a magnetic board, journal, or dedicated notebook to jot down your goals, aspirations, and motivations. Add pictures, key words, or quotes that inspire you. Visualize this vision every day, take a moment to focus on it, and imagine how you will feel when you reach your goals. This visualization practice can fuel your motivation and strengthen your resolve.

- Be kind to yourself:
  Remember that the weight loss journey is a personal one and that each individual has his or her own pace and obstacles to face. Do not seek perfection, but rather progression. Recognize your successes, even the smallest ones, and celebrate every bit of progress you make. Cultivate love and care for yourself, because that is where true long-term motivation comes from.

In addition to lack of motivation, you may also face plateaus during your weight loss program. These periods occur when you experience a lack of progress or a decrease in the rate of weight loss. It can be frustrating and discouraging, but it is important not to give up. Here are some strategies for dealing with plateaus:

- Re-evaluate your habits:
  Consider your workout routine and nutrition. It may be time to make changes or intensify your workout to boost your metabolism. Also evaluate your caloric intake and make sure you are eating enough to support your level of physical activity. You might also consider adding more physical activity into your day, such as taking walks during your lunch break or doing stretching exercises in the morning.

- Add variety to your training:
  If you have noticed a decrease in the rate of weight loss, it may be time to try new workout modalities or new exercises. Adding variety to your workout routine can help break the monotony and stimulate your body in different ways. Try

incorporating new forms of exercise, such as high-intensity cardio, dance, or outdoor activities, to revamp your routine and challenge your body in new ways.

- Pay attention to portion sizes:
  During a plateau, it may be time to review portion sizes. Sometimes, over time, portions can become larger without realizing it. Use measuring cups or a kitchen scale to ensure proper portion sizes and be sure to include a variety of nutritious foods in your diet.

- Take a break and recharge your energy:
  Sometimes, a plateau or lack of motivation can be a sign that you need a break. Don't be afraid to give yourself days off to allow your body to regenerate. Use this time to engage in self-care practices such as adequate rest, active recovery, relaxation techniques such as yoga or meditation, and fulfilling other passions and interests in your life. These breaks can help you regain motivation and renew your dedication to the weight loss journey.

- Maintain patience and perseverance:
  Remember that plateaus are temporary and part of the weight loss journey. Keep patient, be kind to yourself, and continue to follow a healthy routine. Remember that lasting results take time and consistency. Don't let a plateau demotivate you or make you give up on your goals. Keep at it and the results will come with time.

Each individual is unique and you may face specific challenges during your weight loss journey. It is important to tailor the above strategies to your needs and experiment with different solutions to find what works best for you. Never give up, and remember that success requires commitment, perseverance, and a positive mindset.

*When you struggle with lack of motivation, remember that it is a common experience and that you are not alone. I understand that there will be days when the desire to exercise will be minimal and the temptation to quit will be strong. But I invite you to remember why you started this weight loss journey in the first place. Reconnect with that inner flame that drove you to desire positive change in your life. Focus on the deep reasons that motivate you and fuel your determination with a clear vision of your goals.*

*Know that every small step forward counts. Every healthy choice you make, every workout you complete, and every day you stay true to your commitment brings you closer and closer to your goal. Don't underestimate the power of daily actions and the cumulative effect they will have over time. Celebrate every victory, even the smallest, and keep a positive outlook on your progress. Remember that you are on a transformational journey that goes beyond the weight on the scale. It is a journey of self-discipline, resilience, and personal growth.*

*Continue to nurture your inner flame, embrace your inner strength, and recognize the limitless potential within you. Your weight loss journey is an opportunity to transform yourself, not only physically but also mentally and emotionally. Be proud of yourself for embarking on this journey and never lose sight of your goal to be the healthiest, happiest, and most vibrant version of yourself you can be.*

# Time Management

Lack of time is a common challenge many people face when trying to adopt a healthy lifestyle and incorporate an exercise program such as Pilates on a wall. Between work, family, and social responsibilities, it can seem almost impossible to find time to devote to working out and taking care of one's well-being. In this sub-chapter, we will explore issues related to lack and management of time, identify specific challenges that arise, and provide practical solutions to enable you to make time for Pilates on the wall and achieve your goals.

1. **Poor time planning:**
   Organization is the key to optimizing time. Spend time on weekly and daily planning, identifying windows of time in which you can perform Pilates workouts on the wall. Use a planner or time management app to keep track of your schedule and create dedicated workout spaces.

2. **Lack of priority:**
   Set your priorities. Recognize the importance of your own well-being and put Pilates wall exercise at the top of your to-do list. Treat your workout time as a nonnegotiable commitment and keep it consistent. Eliminate activities that are less important or can be delegated to other people to create space for your workout.

3. **Lack of flexibility in the program:**
   Tailor your training program to your needs. Be flexible in choosing the times and days you work out. If your schedule is crowded, consider working out early in the morning or late in the evening. Take advantage of breaks throughout the day to perform short but effective exercises. The important thing is to find a balance that works for you.

4. **Constant interruptions:**
   Eliminate distractions and interruptions during your workout time. Put your phone on silent mode or away from your line of sight. Inform family members or roommates of your workout time so they can respect your privacy and concentration. Create a dedicated workout space that allows you to isolate yourself from outside distractions.

5. **Lack of energy or fatigue:**
   Take care of your body and make sure you get adequate rest and balanced nutrition. Get at least 7–8 hours of sleep per night to replenish your energy. Eat a healthy,

balanced diet that provides you with the nutrients you need to sustain energy during your workout. Avoid excessive consumption of caffeine or refined sugars that can cause energy spikes followed by sudden drops.

6. **Difficulty in managing leisure time:**
Make the most of your free time. Allocate specific time spaces for training and use free time productively. Organize household activities and errands efficiently to free up more time for training. Reduce time spent on social media or watching television and devote that time to your physical well-being.

7. **Feeling of overload or stress:**
Practice stress management techniques such as meditation, deep breathing, or yoga. Set aside time each day to relax and reconnect with yourself. Schedule downtime throughout the day to reduce accumulated stress. Remember that Pilates wall exercise can be an opportunity to release stress and mentally rejuvenate yourself.

8. **Ineffective planning of training sessions:**
Ineffective planning of workouts can undermine desired results. Without a clear structure and defined goals, workouts may be less effective and less motivating. It is important to have strategic planning to maximize the time and energy devoted to Pilates on a wall:

- Set specific goals:
  Before beginning each training session, identify the specific goals you wish to achieve. They might include improving strength, flexibility, posture, or burning calories. Having clear goals will help you focus and organize your exercises accordingly.

- Consult a wall Pilates instructor:
  If you are new to Pilates on a wall or need help planning your workouts, you may want to consult a qualified instructor. An experienced professional can help you create a program tailored to your specific needs and goals.

- Choose the sequence of exercises:
  The sequence of exercises is critical to maximizing the benefits of the workout. Organize the exercises logically, gradually moving from easier to more complex ones. Also consider the involvement of different muscle groups for a complete and balanced workout.

- Consider the duration and frequency of workouts:
  Decide how much time you can devote to workouts and establish a consistent frequency that fits your schedule. Maintain a regularity in your training sessions, whether it's working out every day, three times a week, or according to your needs and availability.

- Keep track of your progress:
  Keep a record of your workouts and the progress you make over time. You can note the exercises you perform, the number of repetitions, the resistance you use, and any other relevant information. This will help you monitor your improvements and adjust your schedule if necessary.

- Take time for recovery:
  Be sure to include recovery periods in your training program. Rest is critical for muscle recovery and injury prevention. To promote recovery and maintain balance in your overall training program, schedule active rest days or devote them to less intense activities, such as stretching or relaxation.

9. **Self-sabotage:**

Self-sabotage in time management can manifest itself through a variety of behaviors that get in the way of achieving your wall Pilates training goals. These behaviors can include procrastination, distractions, lack of prioritization, and lack of discipline. It is important to identify and address these behaviors so that you can manage your time more effectively and dedicate the right amount of time to your workout:

- Identify your habits of self-sabotage: Take time to reflect on your habits and behaviors that lead you to waste time or procrastinate. It can be helpful to keep a journal to identify recurring patterns. Identifying areas where you self-sabotage will help you become aware and take corrective action.

- Develop discipline: Discipline is key to dealing with self-sabotage and managing time effectively. Commit to your training program and adhere to the schedule you set. This will take effort and determination, but once you develop discipline, it will become easier to maintain consistency in training.

- Harness the power of habits: Create habits that support your time management and wall Pilates workout. For example, if you decide to do your workout in the morning, create a routine that includes specific actions to prepare you for your workout, such as putting on your workout clothes and setting up your workout environment. Habits will help you maintain focus and reduce the need to make repeated decisions.

- Make use of time management techniques: Explore different time management techniques to optimize your productivity and reduce wasted time. This can help you maintain focus throughout the day and avoid time wastage.

  One example is the Pomodoro Technique, which involves dividing your work time into sections usually lasting 25 minutes. During each section, you make a concentrated effort to work on a single task without distractions. At the end of the section, you take a short break, usually 5 minutes, to relax and recharge your energy. After every 4 completed sections, you should take a longer break, usually 15–30 minutes.

  This technique helps to improve concentration, combat procrastination, increase time awareness, and promote stress management, plus it can be applied to different aspects of life such as work, home activities, and studying.

- Maintain flexibility: While having a plan and discipline, it is important to maintain flexibility in time management. Life is unpredictable and unforeseen events or emergencies may occur that require flexibility in your training plan. Be kind to yourself and adjust your training plan when necessary, without blaming yourself.

Effective time management is key to integrating Pilates on a wall into your lifestyle and achieving your weight loss goals. Challenge the habits that limit you and take a proactive approach to organizing your time. Remember that devoting time to your well-being is a valuable investment in your long-term health and happiness. Find creative ways to maximize your time and remember that every little bit counts on your path to a healthier, more active life.

# CONCLUSION

Congratulations, dear reader—you have completed your journey toward discovering Pilates on the wall, an art that has the power to transform your approach to fitness and wellness. We hope this book has inspired you and provided you with the knowledge you need to embark on a unique training journey that is challenging, rewarding, and, most importantly, accessible wherever you are.

Pilates on the wall, with its combination of fluid movements, strength, flexibility, and body awareness, offers you an innovative way to achieve your wellness goals. Through the various positions and exercises illustrated, you had the opportunity to discover the incredible potential of your body, experiencing the pleasure of feeling it grow stronger, toned, and more elastic.

Along the way, you learned the importance of listening to your body, understanding the difference between physical hunger and emotional hunger, and dealing with common challenges that can arise along the path to healthy weight loss. We provided you with practical tools to manage time, overcome self-sabotage, and keep motivation alive in achieving your health and fitness goals.

Our intent with this book was to guide you in an empathetic and professional manner, providing an enriching learning experience. We are confident that with the principles of Pilates on the wall and the advice provided, you can embark on a new chapter in your life of wellness, harmony, and self-esteem.

Always remember that the journey to health and wellness is a unique and personal one, and every step forward is an achievement to be celebrated. Whether you are a beginner or a longtime enthusiast, Pilates on the wall offers endless opportunities for growth and discovery.

We encourage you to keep the spirit of enthusiasm alive, to experiment, to explore, and to give yourself the gift of caring for your body and mind. With dedication, perseverance, and the support of Pilates on the wall, you can build a solid foundation for a healthy and happy lifestyle.

Never forget that you are the author of your own story, and this book is just the beginning of an exciting journey that belongs to you. Be kind to yourself, embrace your successes, and welcome challenges with courage. Pilates on the wall will always be here to accompany, support, and inspire you along the way.

Wishing you the utmost success and happiness on your journey to wellness, we greet you with enthusiasm and gratitude.

## BONUS WORKOUT

FRAME THE QRCODE AND DOWNLOAD THE CONTENT. YOU CAN PRINT IT OUT OR KEEP IT ON YOUR PHONE TO CARRY WITH YOU AT ALL TIMES

## WORKOUT PLAYLIST

THIS PLAYLIST IS PERFECT FOR MOTIVATING YOU DURING TRAINING AND GIVING YOU THE RIGHT CHARGE TO OVERCOME YOUR LIMITS

Printed in Great Britain
by Amazon